A Colour Atlas of Clinical Conditions in

Paedodontics

Robert Rapp,
DDS, MS, FRCD(C), FACD

Professor and Chairman
Department of Pedodontics
School of Dental Medicine
University of Pittsburgh
Pittsburgh, Pennsylvania, USA

Chief of Dentistry
Children's Hospital of Pittsburgh
Pittsburgh, Pennsylvania, USA

Gerald B. Winter
MBBS(Lond.), BDS(Lond.), FDS RCS(Eng.), DCH

Professor and Head of Department of
Children's Dentistry, and Sub-Dean
Institute of Dental Surgery
University of London

Hon. Consultant Dental Surgeon
Eastman Dental Hospital
and Queen Elizabeth Hospital for Children
London

Wolfe Medical Publications Ltd
London

The series of Wolfe Medical Atlases brings together probably the world's largest systematic published collection of diagnostic colour photographs.
For a full list of Atlases in the series, including details of our surgical, dental and veterinary Atlases, plus forthcoming titles, please write to Wolfe Medical Publications Ltd, 3–5 Conway Street, London W1.

Published by Wolfe Medical Publications Ltd, 1979
Colour separations by Starf Photolito, Rome
Printed in Italy by Staderini S.p.A.
ISBN 0 7234 0734 7

Contents

To

Connie, Jason, Jordan

and

Eva, Simon, Caroline

Acknowledgements

An Atlas of this nature necessarily draws upon the assistance of many colleagues. Their help, so warmly provided, must be gratefully acknowledged. Due to the limitations imposed by the format of this book, it is not possible to show our indebtedness against each individual illustration; we will therefore list the contributors and indicate which illustrations they have provided for the Atlas: Dr J. O. Andreasen, Mr P. R. Barton **312**, Dr A. Baumhammers **276, 279, 280, 284, 291, 301, 307, 315, 316, 318, 319, 320, 446**, Mr A. H. Brook **466**, Dr M. M. Cohen, Sr. **11, 19, 30, 57, 293, 295, 349, 378, 392, 415, 416, 468, 476, 477**, Mr G. Cross **213, 214, 462**, Dr L. E. Dietz **64**, Dr N. G. El-Labban **326, 327**, Dr W. H. Feasby **444**, Mr M. Geddes **95**, Mr P. D. Gibbard **2**, Dr S. B. Gold and Dr P. Wasserman **50, 51, 225, 333, 422**, Dr J. Guggenheimer **47, 48, 49, 56, 58, 105, 153, 163, 261, 294, 296, 362, 368, 399, 404, 421, 433, 437, 438, 456, 474, 478**, Dr C. W. Hagan **200, 208, 211**, Dr M. I. Houpt **445**, Mr J. D. James **41**, Mr D. Kernohan **366, 410, 411, 461, 472**, Dr A. I. Klein **199**, Mr K. W. Lee **177, 178, 215, 216, 217**, Dr J. R. Mink **346, 467, 475**, Dr S. J. Moss **123**, Dr R. J. Musselman **201**, Dr M. N. Nazif **44**, Mr A. Nesbitt **15, 16, 33, 54, 176, 299, 324, 325, 357, 464**, Mr T. Redpath **385**, Dr V. Rengaswamy **447, 448**, Mr D. C. Rule **338**, Professor G. R. Seward **263**, Mrs Margaret Seward **34**, Dr H. Stein **267**, Dr S. E. Stool **7, 17, 18, 20, 28, 29, 31, 52, 53, 402, 406**, Dr D. A. J. Williamson **457, 458**, Dr G. Z. Wright **113**.

We would also like to give credit to the following institutions which have provided slides for use in this Atlas: Hospital for Sick Children, Toronto, Canada (**45**); Lancaster Cleft Palate Clinic (**372**); University of Pittsburgh Cleft Palate Center (**369, 370, 371**).

In particular we express our gratitude to Mr K. W. Lee for his constructive reading of the manuscript and to Professor R. R. Stephens who initiated the collection of photographic material in the Department of Children's Dentistry, Institute of Dental Surgery, London.

The following Journals and persons are credited and given thanks for allowing reproduction of previously published illustrations:

1. Archives of Disease in Childhood and Dr M. J. Simpkiss **285, 286, 470**
2. Churchill Livingstone and Mr J. C. Mustardé **240, 242, 350, 365, 384, 396, 439, 440**
3. British Dental Journal **2, 92, 130, 165, 166, 212, 317, 473**
4. Journal of Dentistry for Children and Dr J. R. Mink **346, 467**, Dr M. M. Cohen, Sr. **293, 392**
5. W. B. Saunders Co. **75, 76, 98, 126, 146, 156, 157, 158, 162, 167, 442, 463**
6. Baillière Tindall **104, 193, 336, 358, 360, 394**
7. Academic Press and Dr M. M. Breuer **170, 193**

The skilled assistance and technical advice of the following people must be acknowledged: Mr W. J. Morgan, Photographic Department, Institute of Dental Surgery, University of London and Mr J. R. Gibel and Mr H. E. Sweitzer, Photographic Department, School of Dental Medicine, University of Pittsburgh.

Mrs Mary Kuhn of the University of Pittsburgh and Miss Elaine Harwood of the University of London must both receive special recognition for their tireless assistance not only in typing manuscripts but also in tending to the multitude of details that become so important while preparing the manuscript for the publisher.

Introduction

This Atlas is a collection of clinical and radiographic illustrations depicting oral and related diseases and anomalies which have been observed in our patients and patients of many of our colleagues. Our objective in preparing this book is to provide clinicians and students with an easily usable reference tool to assist in the recognition and diagnosis of such conditions.

An Atlas of this type is not a textbook and therefore is not meant to be thoroughly comprehensive. Descriptions of the normal may be found elsewhere and no further duplication is intended here. This Atlas elects solely to illustrate a series of abnormal conditions with some of their variations. The format and size of the book preclude presentation of treatment.

As this Atlas is designed to serve as a consultative source for the types of disease and abnormality mentioned above, the reader may benefit from a description of its organisation. The opening chapter is subdivided into sections listed under the principle anatomical features of the head; the following five chapters deal separately with the intraoral structures; the penultimate chapter covers the problems related to the jaws, and the final chapter concerns the limbs. This last chapter may appear out of place in an Atlas devoted to conditions in paedodontics, but the intention is to limit the illustrations to conditions already dealt with or closely related to those described elsewhere in the book. It is our belief that a general examination of the patient may assist in establishing a diagnosis for an otherwise puzzling condition, and that the limbs are the most accessible portions of the body for this purpose. An anatomical 'regionalisation' of this type may also be of assistance to the busy clinician who, when confronted with an unusual condition, need only consult the chapter appropriate to the part concerned to establish a diagnosis. Such an approach, however, is not meant to minimise the importance of a thorough history, detailed clinical and radiographic examinations and, when appropriate, a biopsy.

The authors feel their efforts will be amply rewarded if this Atlas helps to expedite the recognition of diseases or abnormalities in our young patients.

1. The cranium and face

a. Cranium

1

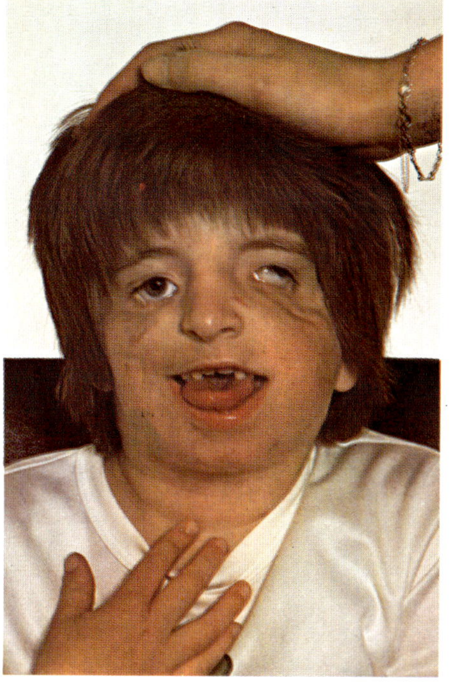

1 Mandibulofacial dysostosis (Treacher Collins syndrome) Marked facial deformity in a 6 year old boy with typical antimongoloid obliquity of the palpebral fissures due to maxillary and zygomatic bony hypoplasia; micrognathia of the mandible; bilateral deformity of the pinnae with atresia of the external auditory meati; severe subnormality and a cleft of the secondary (posterior) palate. Sielastic implants have been inserted into the cheeks in an attempt to improve facial appearance.

2

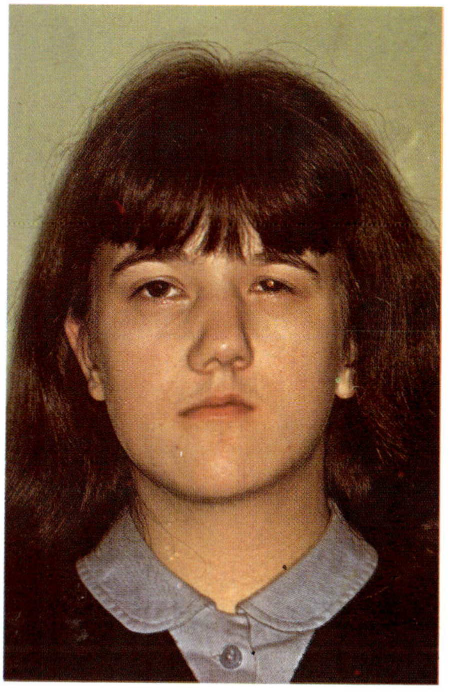

2 Unilateral facial hypoplasia The soft tissues and bone on the left side of the face are markedly underdeveloped in this 13 year old girl. The cause is unknown and there is no family history. A generalised irregular microdontia of permanent teeth displaying enamel hypoplasia is associated with the facial deformity.

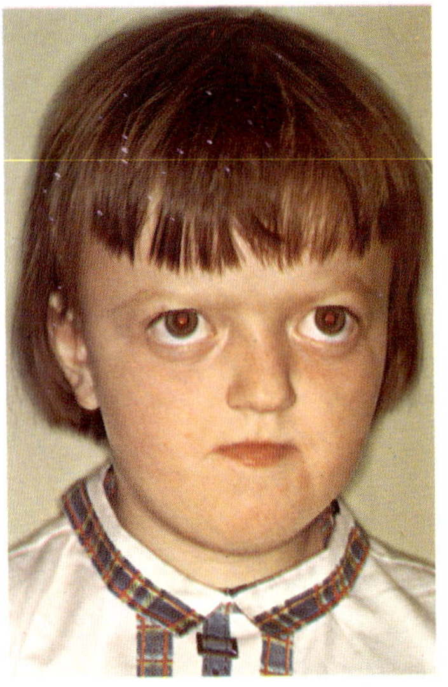

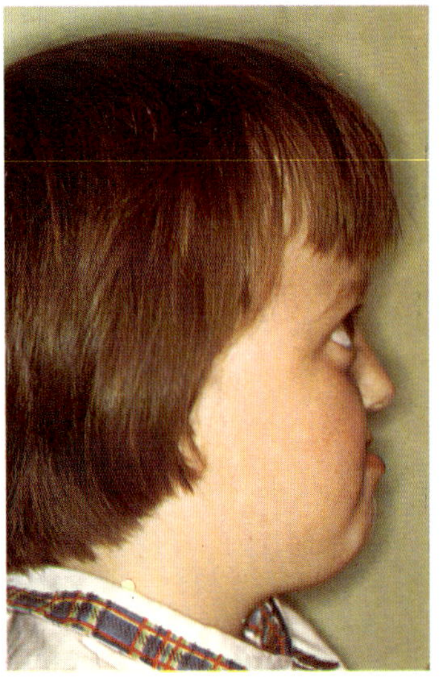

3, 4 Craniofacial dysostosis (Crouzon's syndrome) The malformations of the face and skull in this 3 year old girl are due to the premature fusion of the cranial sutures associated with maxillary hypoplasia. Bilateral proptosis, maxillary retrognathia and a beak nose are all typical features of this syndrome.

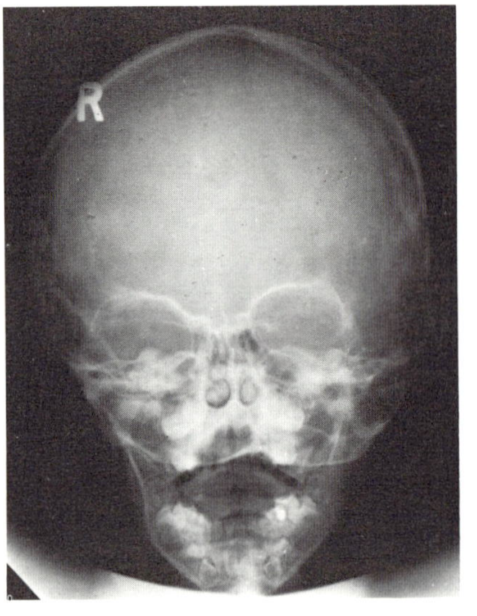

5, 6 Radiographs of the child seen in **3** and **4** show the characteristic premature synostosis of the coronal and sagittal sutures and the 'copper beaten' appearance of the calvarium due to the increased digital markings.

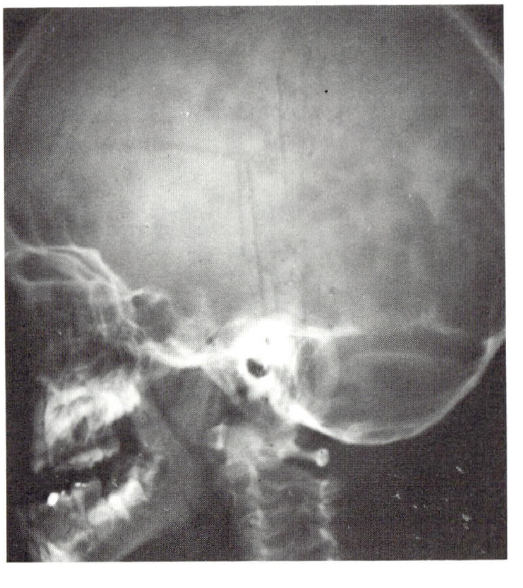

7 Acrocephalosyndactyly (Apert's syndrome) The characteristic facial appearance of Apert's syndrome is seen in this boy with a high towering forehead, small beak-like nose and a tendency to proptosis. Premature fusion of a number of cranial sutures, especially the coronal, and maxillary hypoplasia are also seen in this condition which is frequently associated with mental subnormality. (See **378** and **476**)

7

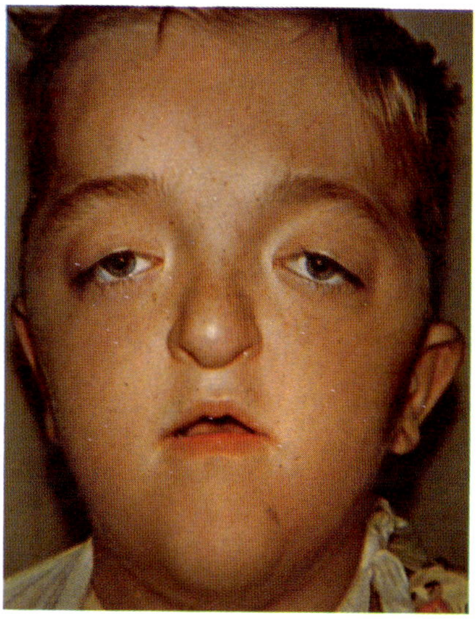

8, 9 Cleidocranial dysostosis Radiographs of 10 year old boy with cleidocranial dysostosis. Note retrognathic maxilla, persistence of many cranial sutures, numerous Wormian bones in the region of the lambdoidal suture, bitemporal bossing and multiple supernumerary teeth in the anterior portions of the maxilla and mandible. (See **79**)

8

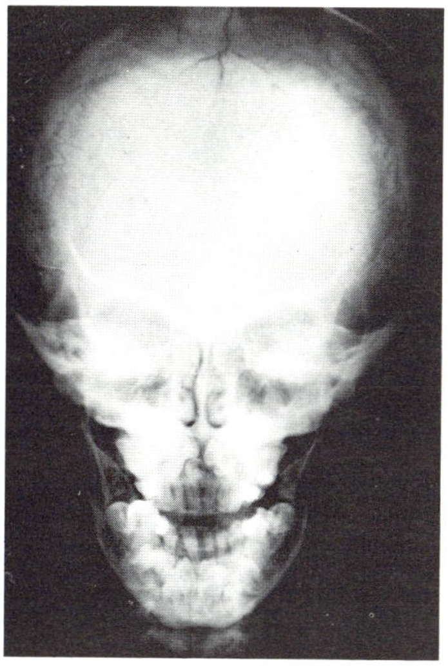

9

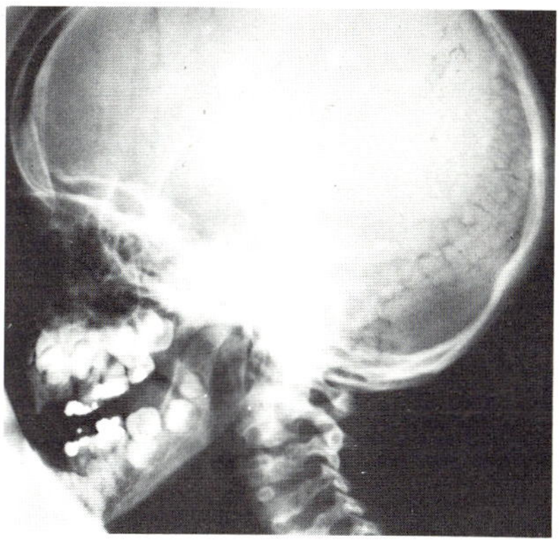

10 Almost total absence of clavicles can be seen in this chest radiograph of the case seen in **8** and **9**.

10

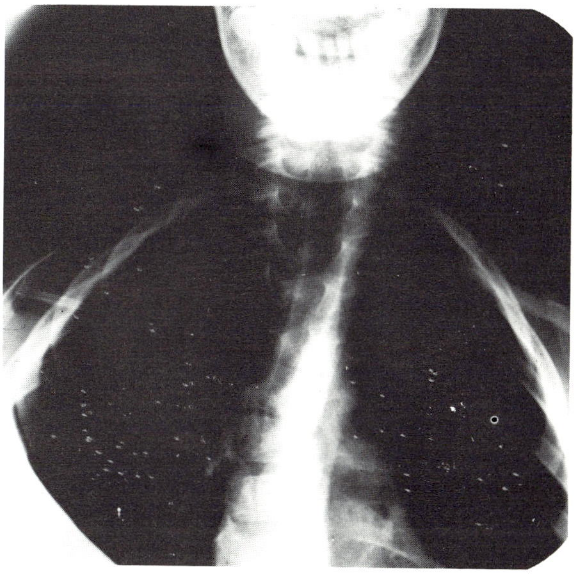

11 Hydrocephalus The abnormal accumulation of cerebro-spinal fluid intracranially at an early age led to the enlarged cranium in this 7 year old boy with hydrocephalus.

11

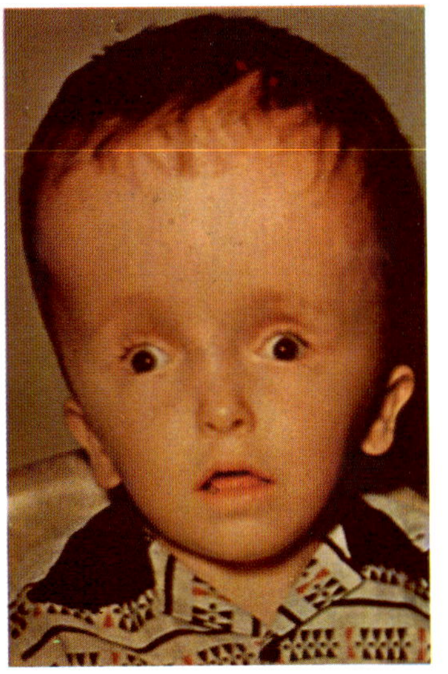

b. Face

(i) General

12, 13 Hemifacial hypoplasia (First Arch syndrome) Structures developed from the first branchial arch are defective in this 8 year old boy. Such defects are manifested by hypoplasia of the left side of the mandible, the left maxilla and zygomatic bones, malformation of the left pinna (which has already undergone plastic surgery) and atresia of the external auditory meatus.

12

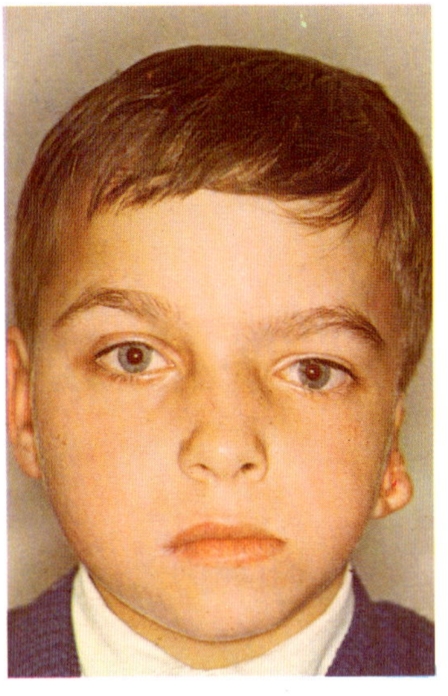

13

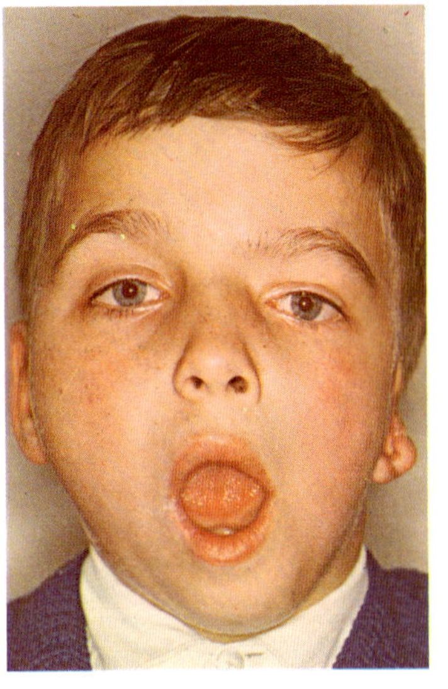

14 Radiograph of the child shown in **12** and **13**.

14

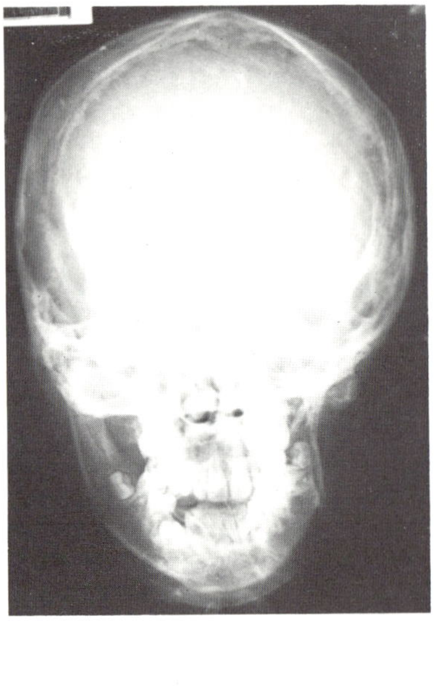

15

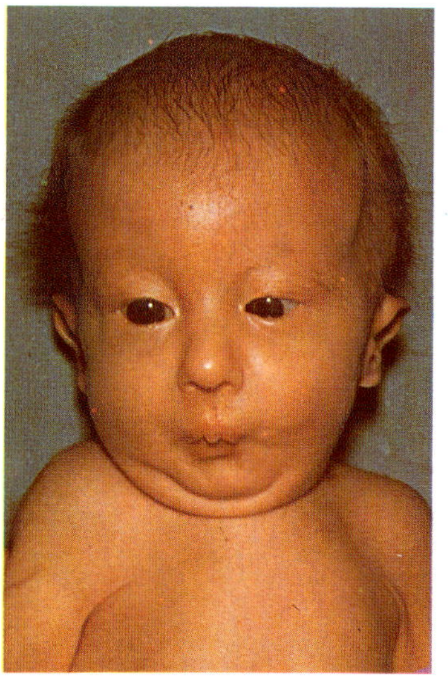

15, 16 Pierre Robin syndrome The severe mandibular micrognathia characteristic of the Pierre Robin syndrome is seen in this affected infant. The other manifestations of the condition are a cleft of the secondary (posterior) palate and glossoptosis.

16

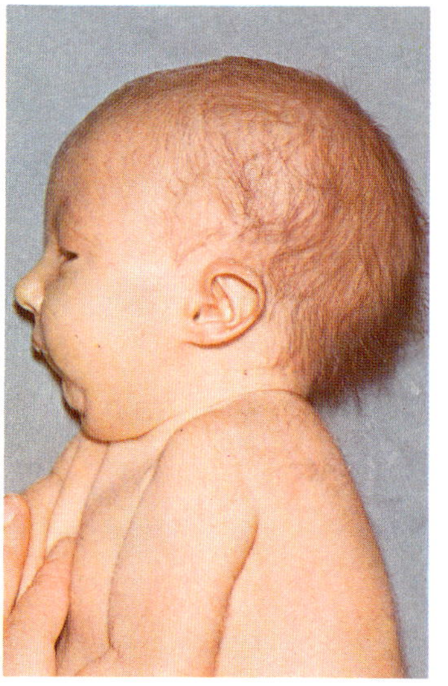

17

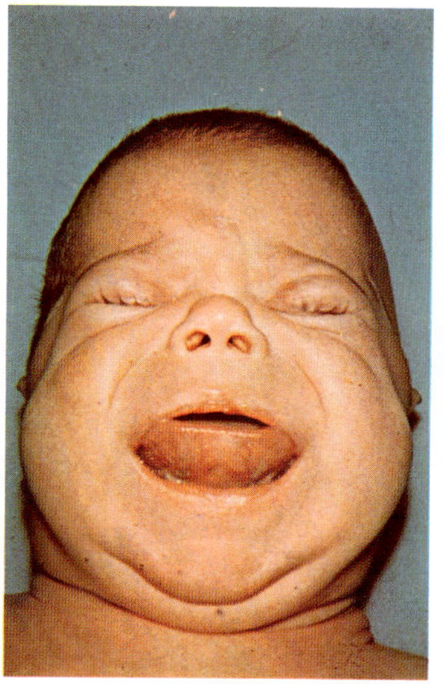

17 Congenital hypothyroidism (Cretinism) This infant with cretinism or congenital hypothyroidism has the classical features of puffiness about the eyes, large protruding tongue and sparse dry hair.

18

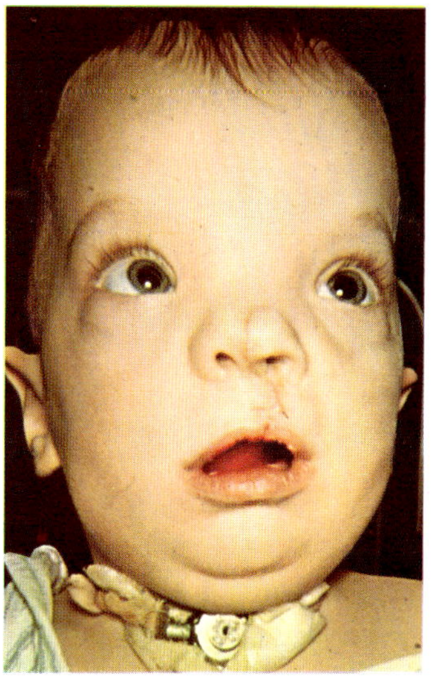

18 Hypertelorism Hypertelorism, as seen in this infant, is characterised by an abnormally large distance between the pupils of the eyes and a flattening of the bridge of the nose. Mental retardation is more common in children with hypertelorism than in the normal population. The tracheostomy was required for postoperative complications after a repair of the cleft lip and palate.

19 Trisomy 13–15 syndrome (Patau's syndrome) Bilateral cleft lip and palate as seen in this infant with Patau's syndrome is a nearly constant feature of this chromosomal anomaly. Other signs are microcephaly and low-set ears.

19

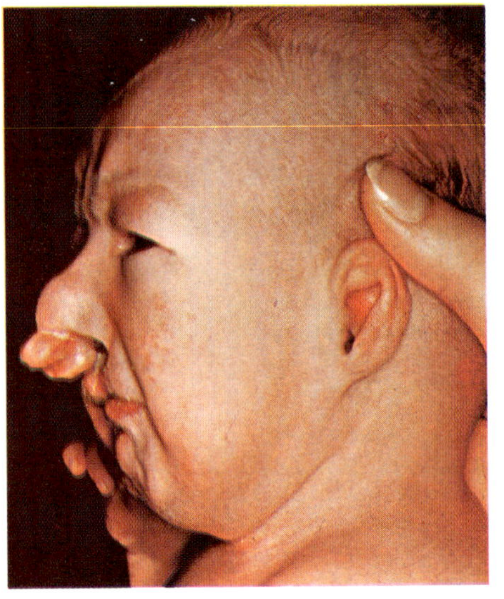

20 Oculoauriculovertebral dysplasia (Goldenhar's syndrome) Several of the facial features of Goldenhar's syndrome are present in this affected infant. In particular the ocular dermoid and the pedunculated auricular appendix are two common findings. The bilateral cleft lip and palate are less constant features of the syndrome.

20

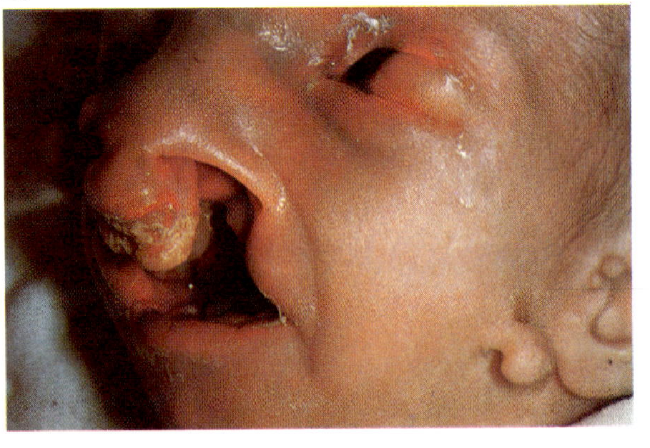

21 Down's syndrome (Mongolism, Trisomy 21) The underdevelopment of the middle third of the face with relative mandibular prognathism is seen in this adolescent with Down's syndrome. The open mouth posture with the obvious presence of a relatively large tongue is another feature of this chromosomal anomaly.

21

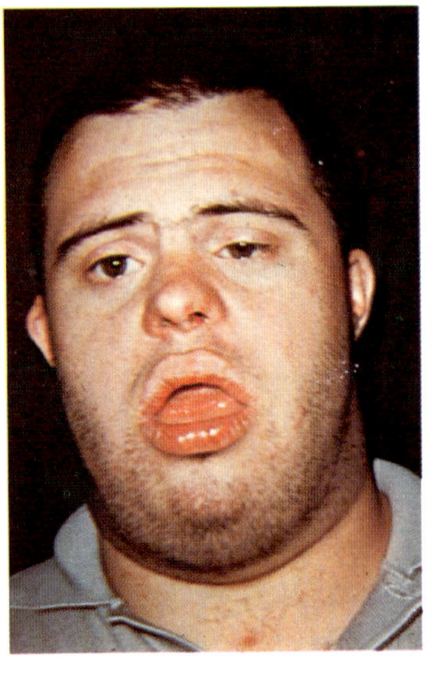

22, 23 Hypohidrotic ectodermal dysplasia The obvious sparsity of scalp hair and deficiency of eyebrows and eyelashes in this 13 year old boy with X-linked recessive hypohidrotic ectodermal dysplasia are typical of the syndrome. Other features of the condition are the protruberant lips and the outstanding ears. (See **90** and **91**)

22

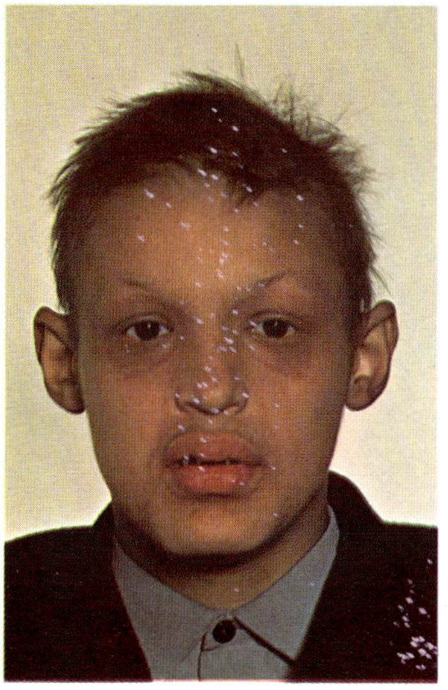

23

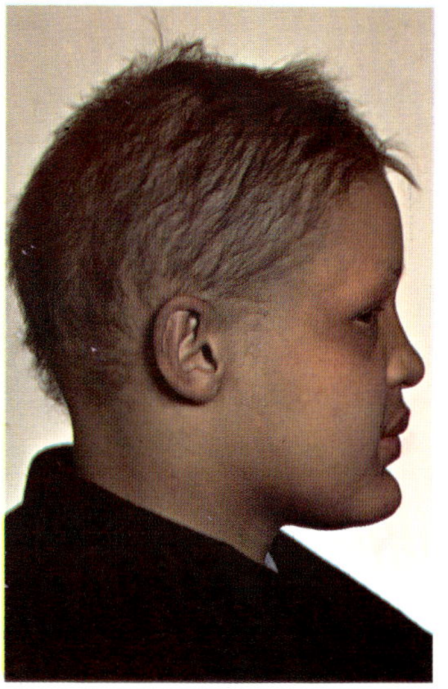

24 Ectodermal dysplasia The gross deficiency of eyebrows and eyelashes is the principal facial feature of an autosomal dominant form of ectodermal dysplasia in this 10 year old girl. Her mother and maternal grandmother were similarly affected. (See **92**)

24

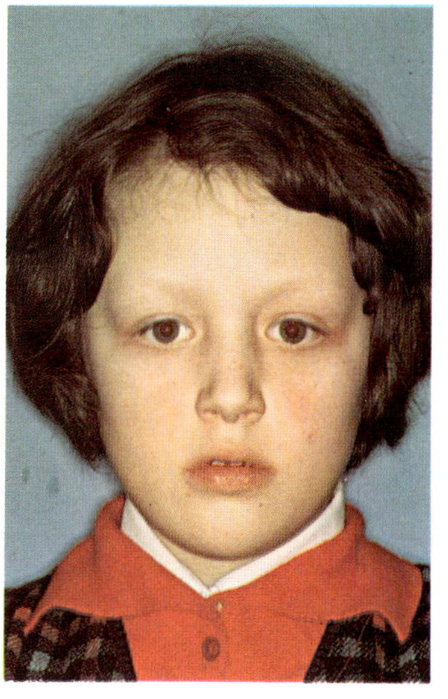

25 Facial palsy (Bell's palsy) When asked to smile this 11 year old girl is unable to elevate the left side of the upper lip, giving evidence of a lower motor neurone paralysis of the facial (VIIth) nerve on this side of her face. She also suffers from a loss of taste on the left side of the anterior portion of the tongue.

25

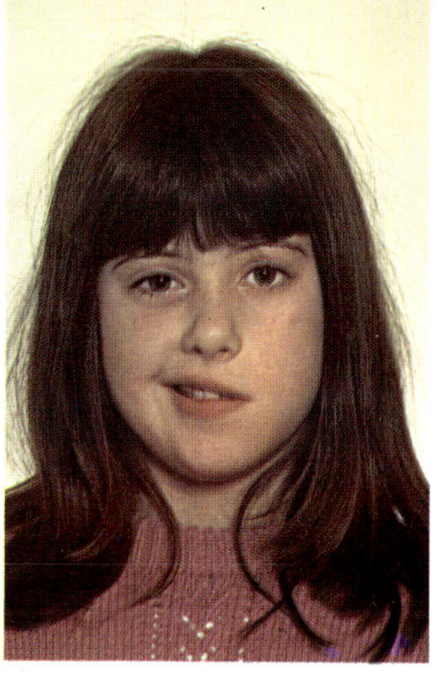

26 Capillary haemangioma (Port-wine stain, Naevus flammeus) The left side of the face in this young girl is disfigured by an extensive capillary haemangioma or port-wine stain. (See **303**)

26

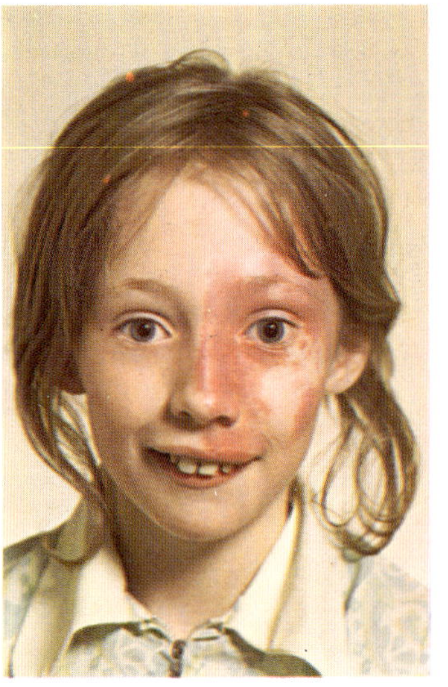

27 Cavernous haemangioma The facial asymmetry in this adolescent boy is due to the presence on the left side of a deep seated and extensive cavernous haemangioma. Hamartomatous malformations of this type usually continue to enlarge during the normal period of bodily growth and then cease to develop further. (See **384**)

27

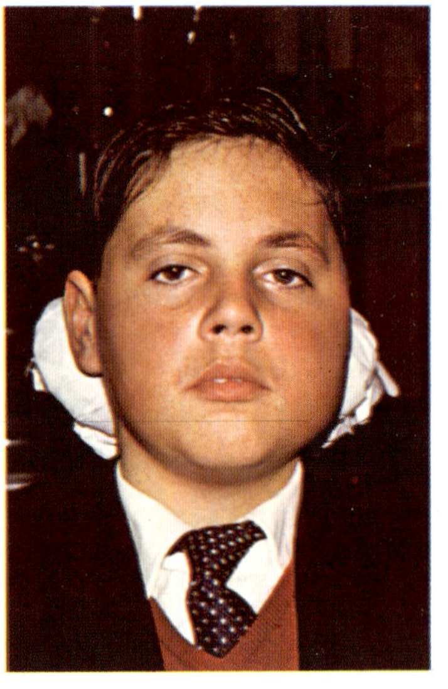

28 Neurofibroma The unilateral periorbital and facial swelling in this infant is due to extensive involvement of the tissues by a neurofibroma. Total surgical excision of these lesions cannot be undertaken and malignant change occasionally occurs in later life.

28

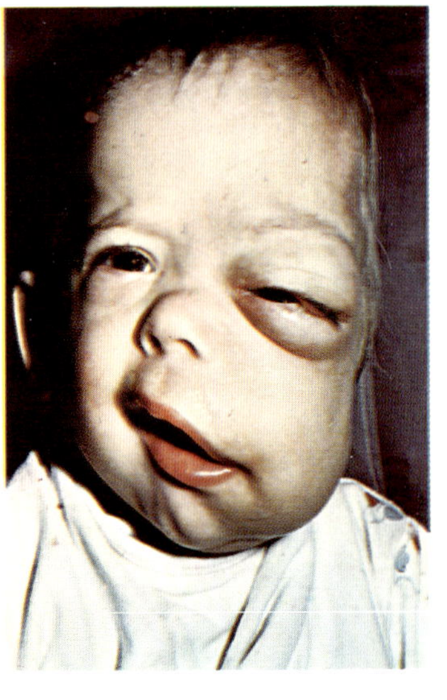

29 Neuroblastoma Neuroblastoma of the adrenal gland is one of the common malignant tumours of infancy. This affected young child with bilateral orbital swelling demonstrates a frequent site for metastatic spread of the tumour.

29

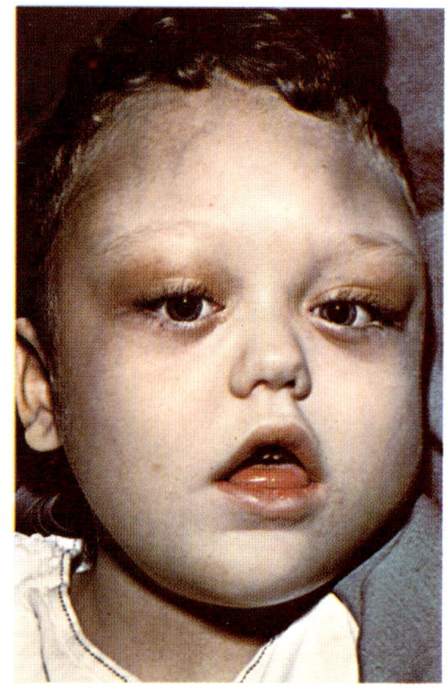

30 Tuberous sclerosis (Epiloia) The facial skin in this 15 year old boy is widely involved by a large number of small, reddish angiofibromatous lesions, some of which are raised above the surface. Similar lesions are present on the skin of the trunk and other parts of the body. An associated moderate mental retardation indicates involvement of the central nervous system.

30

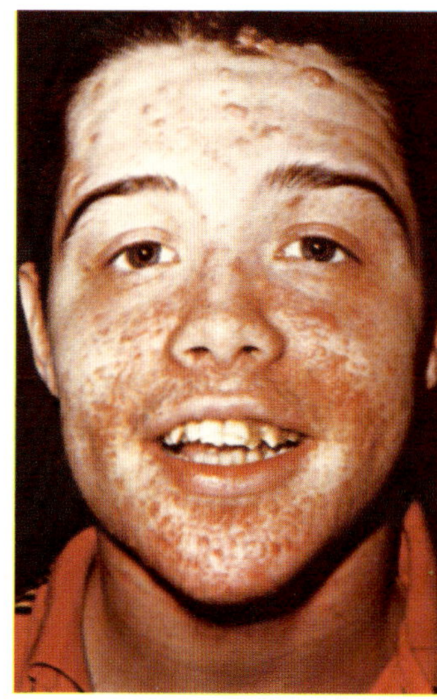

31 Acute suppurative parotitis (Parotid abscess) Acute infections of the parotid gland by Staphylococcus aureus are frequently complicated by abscess formation. This girl has an abscess of the right parotid gland which is draining through a sinus in the region of the gonial angle. Infections of this type are mainly confined to individuals suffering from extreme debility.

31

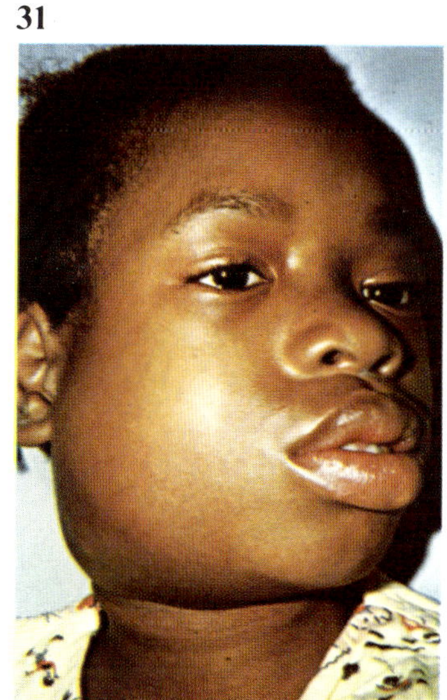

32

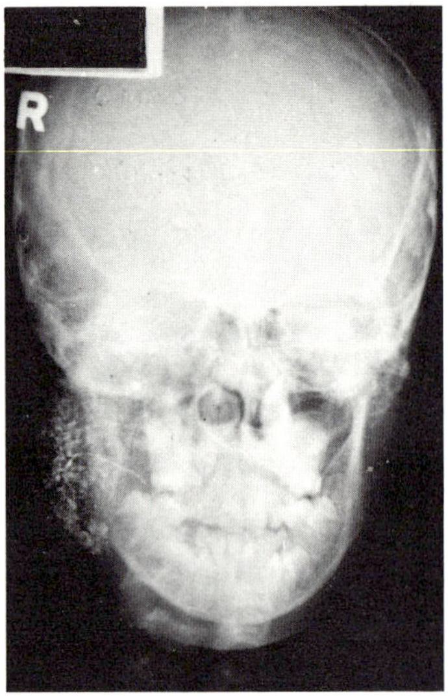

32 Recurrent subacute parotitis A sialogram of the right parotid gland is shown in this radiograph of an 11 year old girl with a history of recurrent subacute parotitis. Numerous small collections of radiopaque media can be seen which demonstrate the presence of sialectasis. The infective organism in such cases is generally Streptococcus viridans.

33

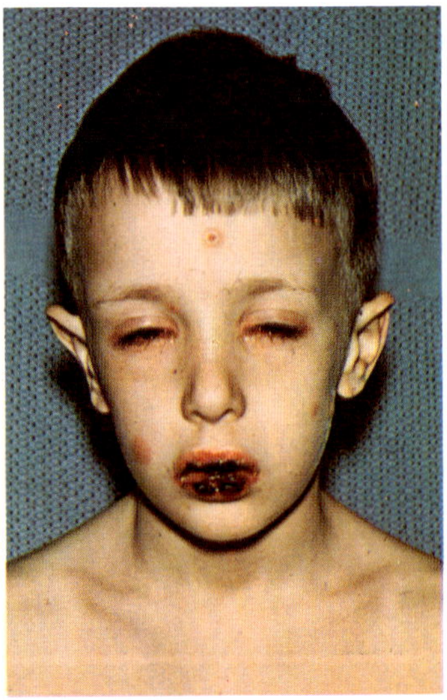

33 Erythema multiforme exudativum (Stevens-Johnson syndrome) An obviously ill boy with the severe mucosal changes of erythema multiforme exudativum affecting the conjunctival and oral tissues. The typical 'target' appearance of the skin lesions can be seen on the forehead and right cheek.

(ii) Cheeks

34

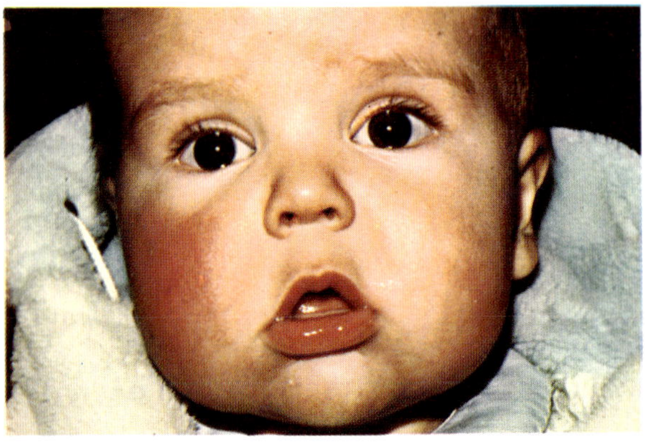

34 Cheek flush Unilateral hyperaemia or flushing of the cheek as seen in this infant is frequently associated with the process of teething. The eruption of the primary molars is responsible for cheek flushing more frequently than the emergence of the anterior teeth.

35 Facial cellulitis The bright redness of the left cheek is associated with redness and swelling of the lower eyelid in this young girl. The inflammation is due to a spreading infection through the facial tissues originating from a dentoalveolar abscess on a cariously exposed maxillary primary canine.

35

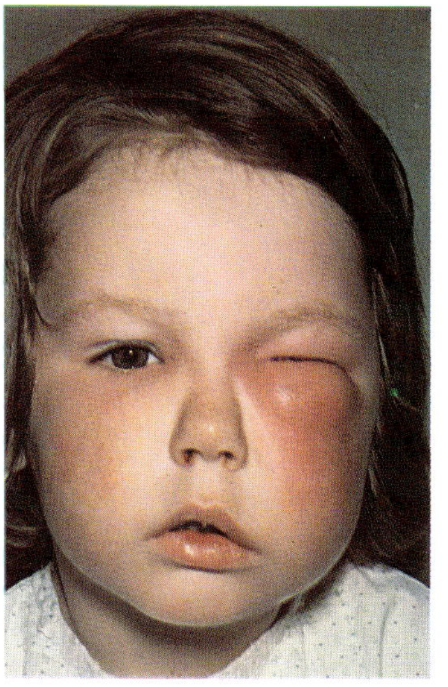

36

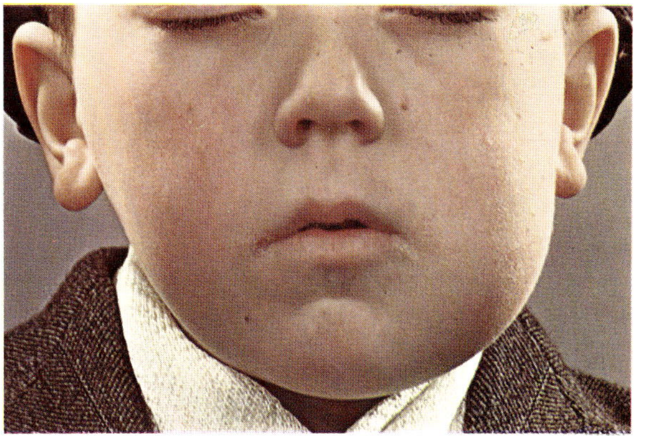

36 Dentoalveolar abscess The swelling of the left cheek in this boy is due to a dentoalveolar abscess on a cariously exposed mandibular primary molar. The swelling has been present for a week.

37 Lymphangioma The involvement of the right cheek by a lymphangiomatous malformation is responsible for considerable facial deformity in this 6 year old boy. (See **350**)

37

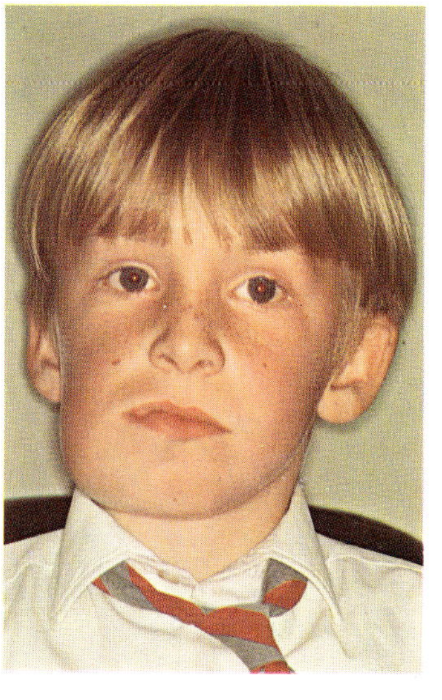

38

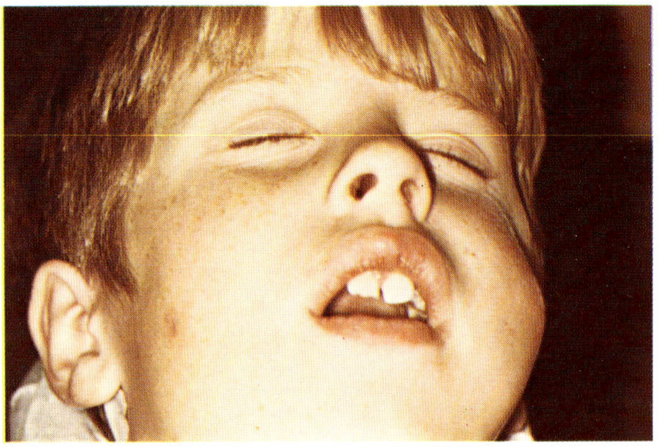

38 Haematoma The left cheek of this boy is swollen by a large haematoma resulting from a posterior superior alveolar nerve block.

39

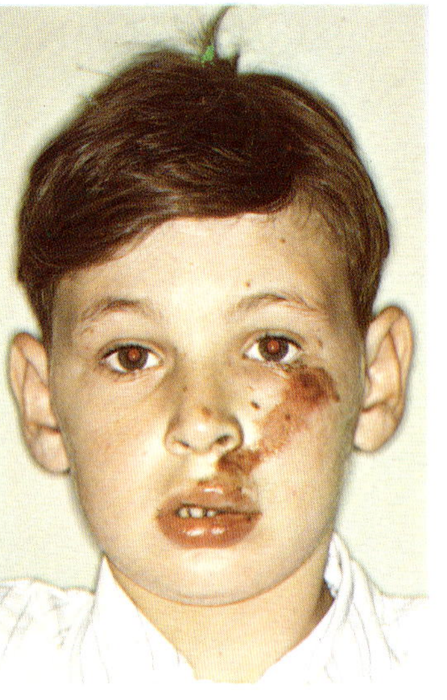

39 Facial abrasion Facial trauma from a bicycle accident has resulted in severe abrasions of the left cheek and upper lip in this 10 year old boy. (See **237** and **238**)

40

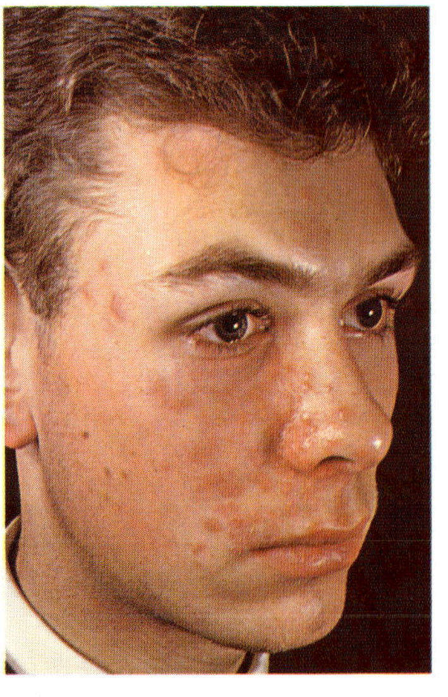

40 Herpes zoster The lesions of herpes zoster are mainly limited to the distribution of the second (maxillary) division of the trigeminal (Vth) nerve on the right side of the face in this adolescent boy. One or two isolated lesions affecting the first (ophthalmic) division may be seen in the forehead over the right eye. (See **289** and **389**)

41 Cancrum oris Gross destruction of the cheek and underlying bony tissues of the maxilla and mandible from cancrum oris is seen in this young Nigerian child. The condition has been arrested with antibiotic treatment. Persistent drooling of saliva is present through the facial defect.

41

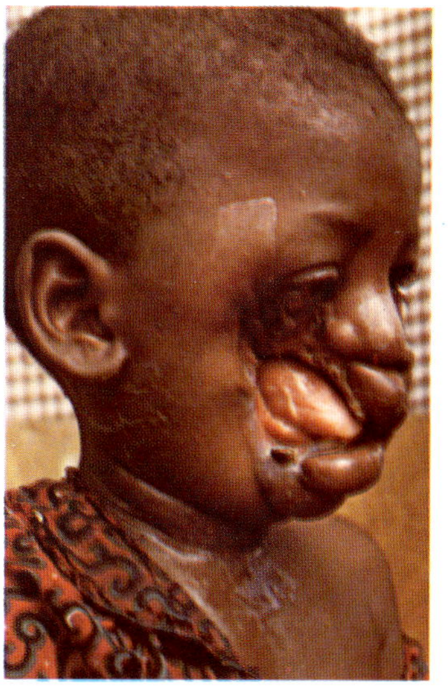

(iii) Nose

42, 43 Unilateral cleft lip and palate A 'dish-faced' deformity of the middle third of the face is evident in this 7 year old girl with a repaired unilateral cleft lip and palate. Also evident is the typical flattening of the left side of the nose on the side of the lip repair. (See **425** and **426**)

42

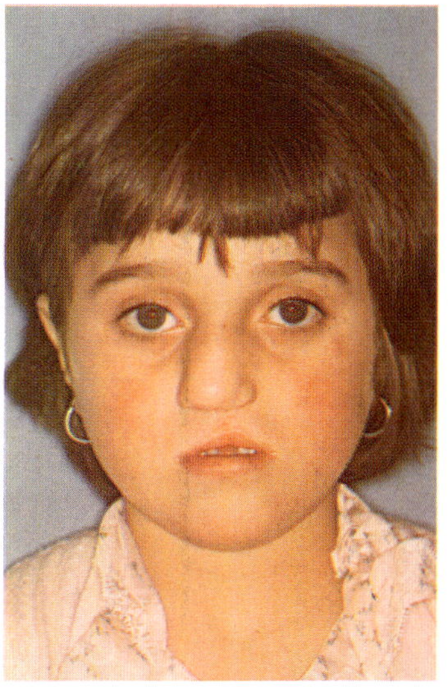

43

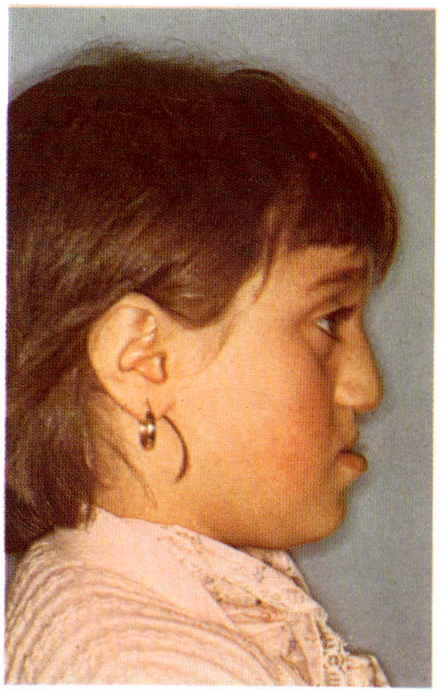

44 Foreign body in nasal passage A dislodged rubber dam clamp is visible in the nasopharynx in this radiograph of a young child.

44

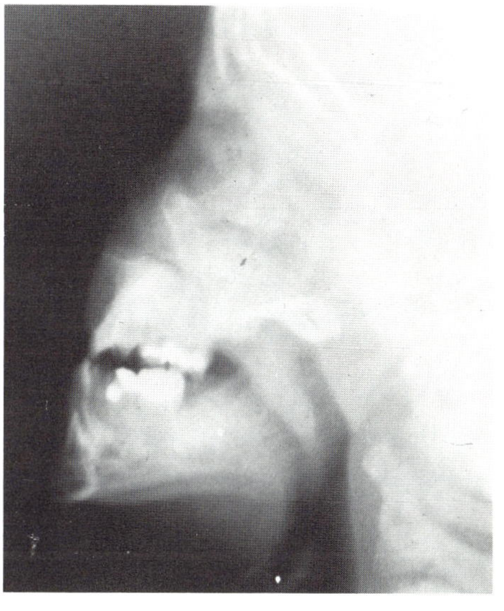

(iv) Lips

45

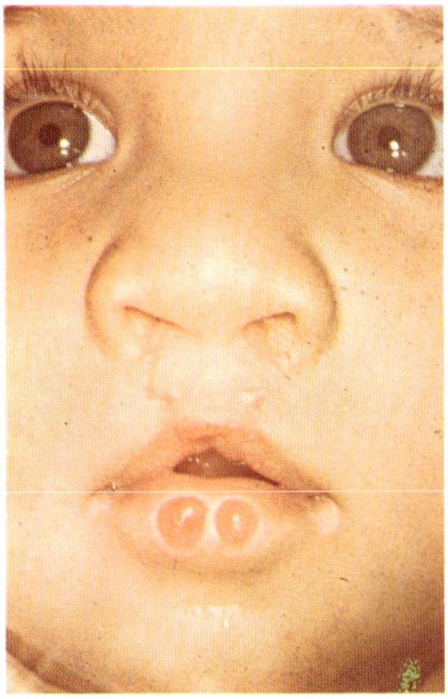

45 Lip-pit syndrome Two congenital pits are located on either side of the midline of the lower lip in this infant with a repaired bilateral cleft of lip and palate. Abnormalities of the extremities have been noted in association with this syndrome.

46

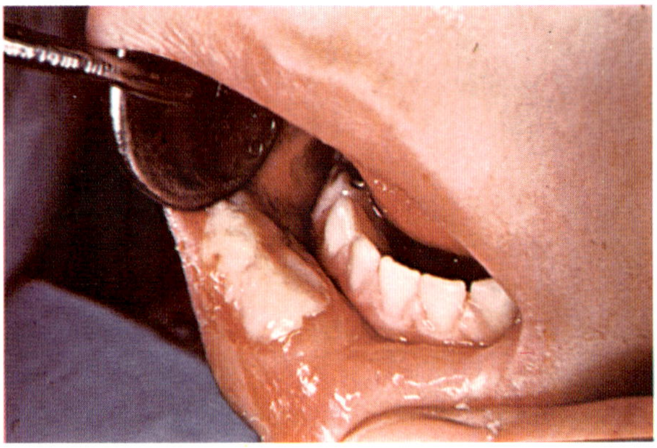

46 Lip trauma A whitened area of mucosal sloughing surrounded by a bright red margin of erythema is present on the right side of the lower lip. The lesion was produced by biting the tissues which had been anaesthetised with a mandibular nerve block.

47

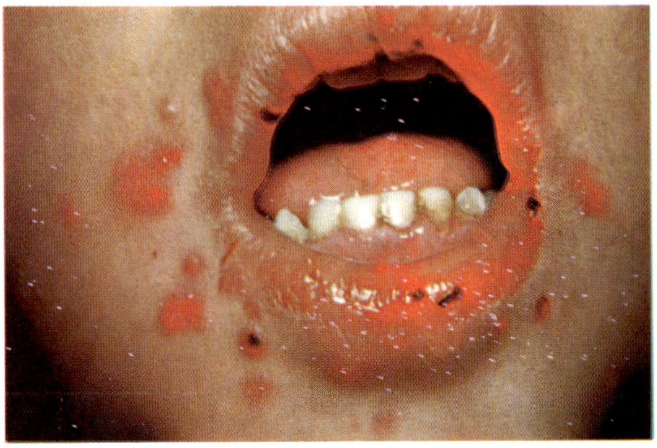

47 Acute herpetic infection This young child has an acute primary infection by the herpes simplex virus. Vesicular and ulcerated lesions can be seen on the mucosa of the lips, at the mucocutaneous (vermilion) border and on the facial skin.

48

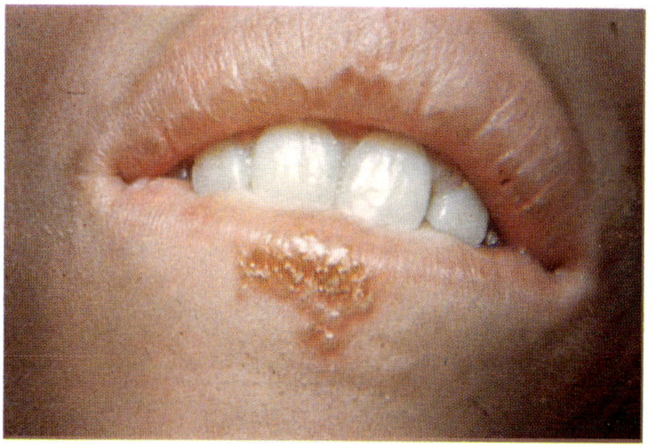

48 Herpes labialis A crop of vesicles at the mucocutaneous border of the lower lip denotes a recurrence of herpes simplex virus infection in this child.

49

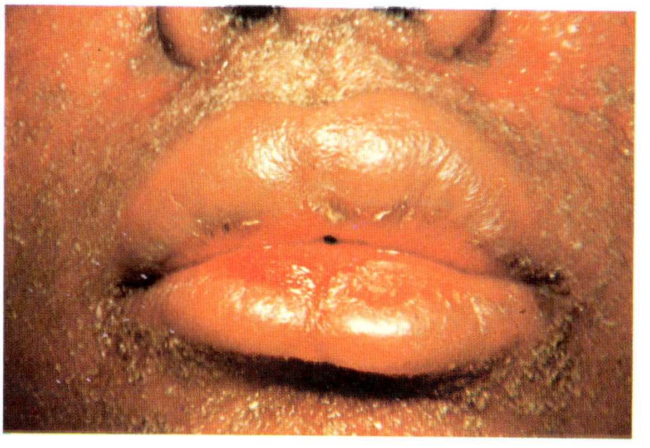

49 Penicillin hypersensitivity (allergy) This boy displays swollen lips and a scaly dermatitis of the facial skin as a result of a severe allergic reaction to systemically administered penicillin.

50

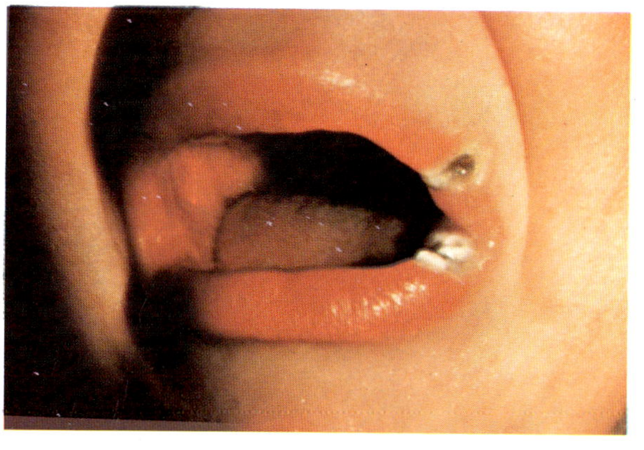

50 Electrical burn At the age of 18 months this child sustained burns of the lips from chewing a live electrical cord.

51

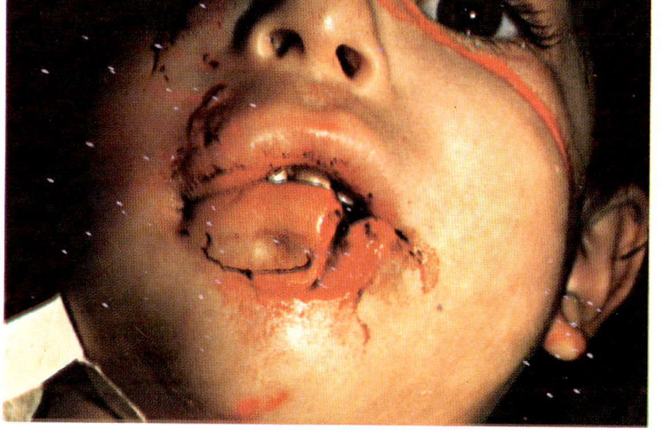

51 Facial lacerations An attack by a watch-dog on this 3 year old boy produced multiple facial lacerations including a severe full-thickness tear of the lower lip.

52

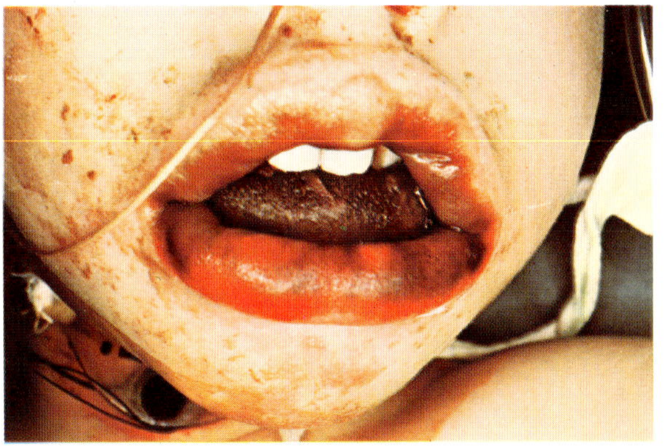

52 Caustic burns The ingestion of a caustic substance was responsible for the severe burns to the face, lips and mouth in this child. A tracheostomy was required to maintain respiration.

53

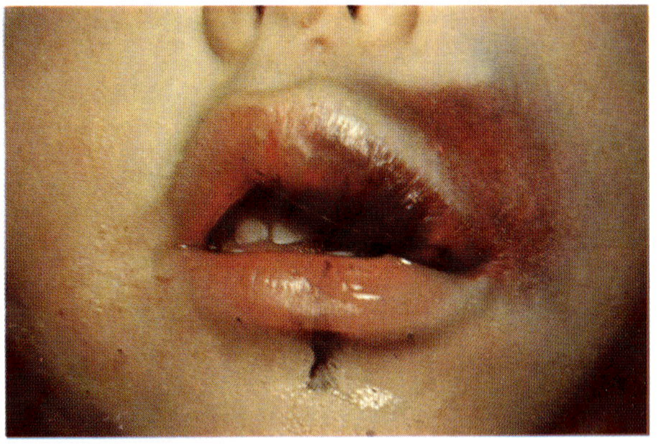

53 Haematoma This haemophiliac child has a large haematoma of the upper lip and face.

(v) Eyes

54

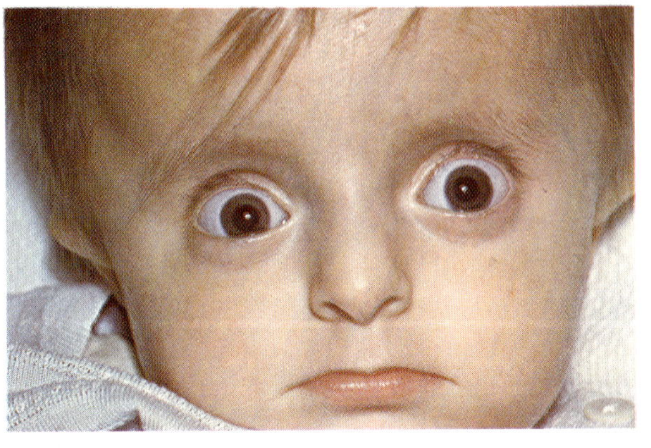

54 Osteogenesis imperfecta This infant with osteogenesis imperfecta shows the characteristic marked blueness of the sclerae. Note also the bitemporal bossing of the skull seen in this condition. (See **176** and **477**)

55

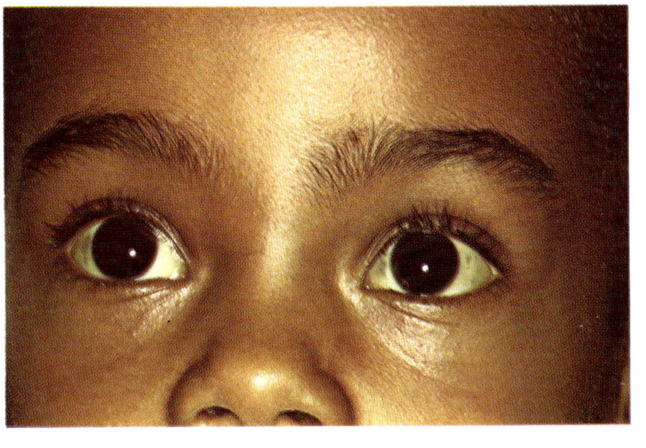

55 Sickle cell anaemia The yellow tinge to the sclerae of this 4 year old girl is due to the presence of jaundice (hyperbilirubinaemia), frequently associated with sickle cell anaemia. (See **302**)

56 Exophthalmos The protruding eyes of this boy are characteristic of the exophthalmos associated with hyperthyroidism.

56

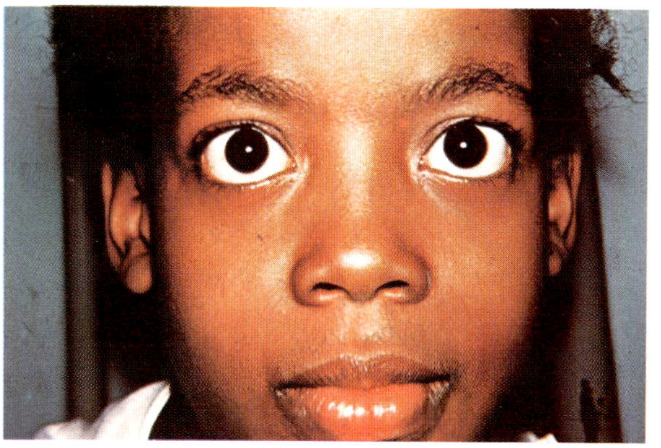

57 Encephalofacial angiomatosis (Sturge-Weber syndrome) The presence of a large cavernous haemangioma near the outer margin of the right eye in this child with the Sturge-Weber syndrome gives the appearance of a double eye.

57

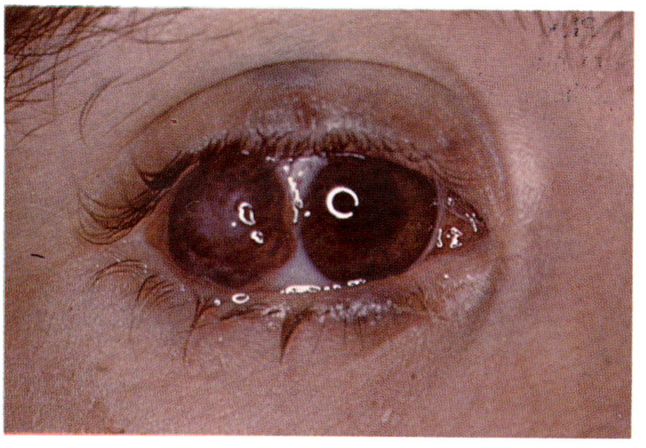

58 Acute herpetic infection Acute primary infection of the conjunctiva by the herpes simplex virus is responsible for the redness, lacrimation and photophobia in this young child.

58

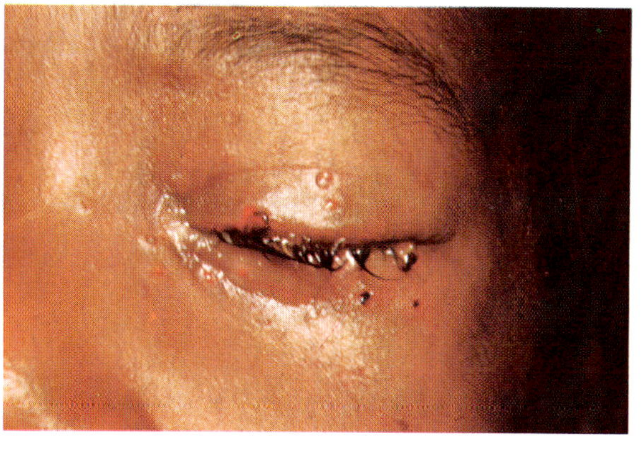

(vi) Chin

59 Acute dentoalveolar abscess The bright redness and swelling at the front of the chin in this teenage boy are due to the pointing of a dentoalveolar abscess from a previously traumatised mandibular permanent central incisor.

59

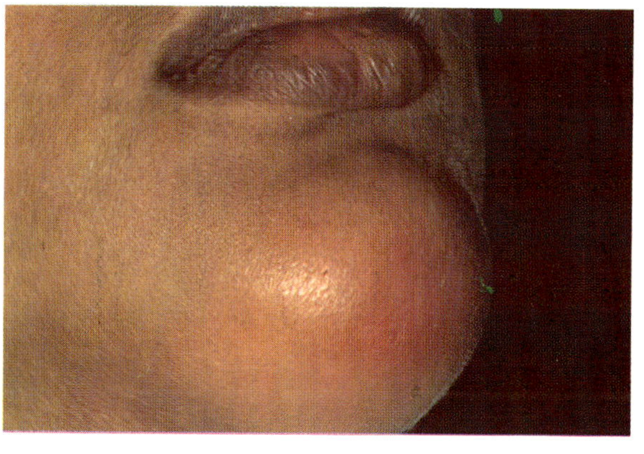

60 Submandibular sinus The sinus present on the skin in the left submandibular region of this 3 year old girl has been caused by the local application of heat to an underlying abscess causing it to burst. The abscess was derived from an acute suppurative infection of the submandibular lymph nodes.

60

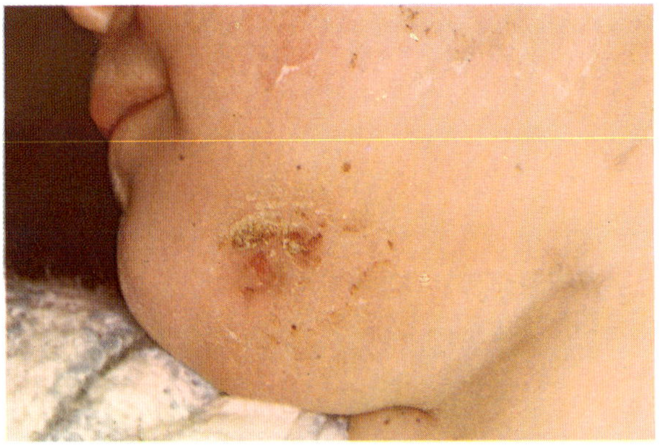

61 Plexiform neurofibromatosis The café-au-lait pigmentation of the skin overlying the chin, together with the swelling of the subcutaneous and mucosal tissues on the left side of the face suggested the diagnosis of neurofibromatosis in this 11 year old boy. Subsequent biopsy showed the lesion to have characteristic histological appearances of a plexiform neurofibroma. (See **313** and **314**)

61

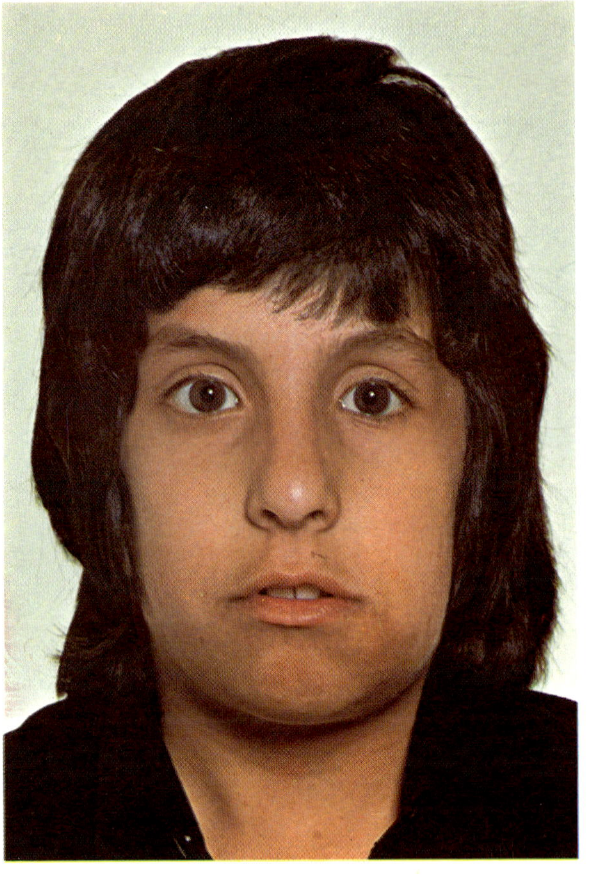

2. The teeth

a. Number

(i) Supernumerary teeth

62

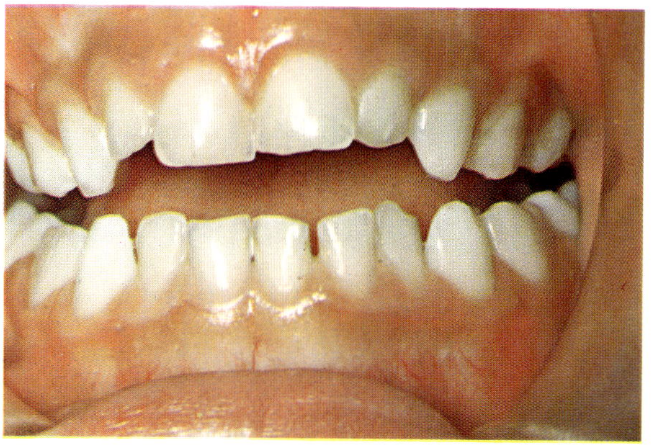

62 Supplemental primary incisor An extra incisor is present in the mandibular labial segment. Due to the normal shape of all these incisors, it is difficult to identify the extra tooth.

63

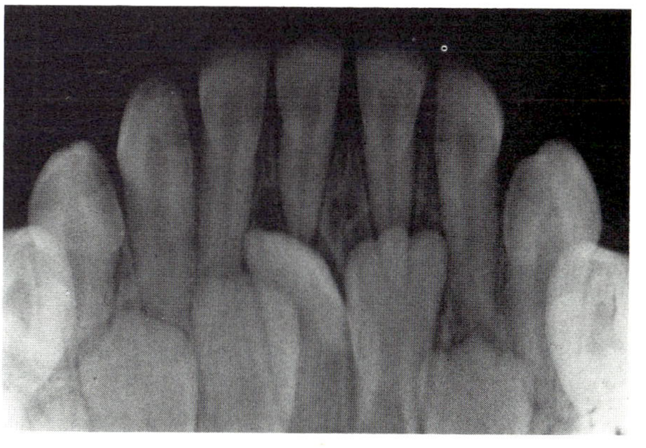

63 Supernumerary primary incisor Conical supernumerary primary incisor shown in radiograph of mandibular labial segment. A permanent supernumerary successor lying beneath can also be seen.

64

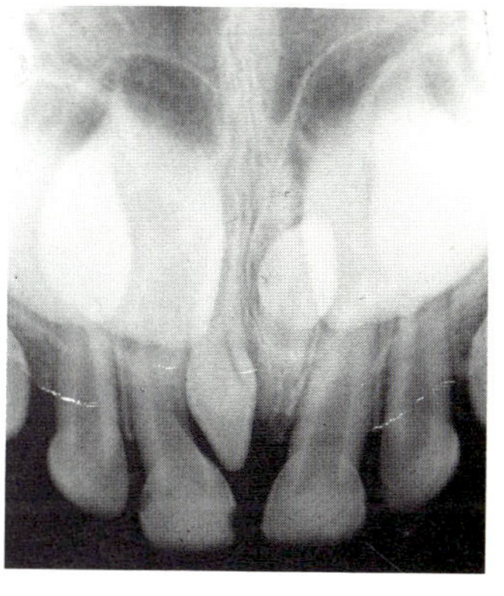

64 Bilateral mesiodens Bilateral mesiodens shown in radiograph of the premaxillary region; the left mesiodens is inverted.

65, 66 Mesiodens Conical mesiodens which has erupted palatally to the maxillary central incisors. Unless extracted early it is disfiguring and may interfere with the occlusion.

65

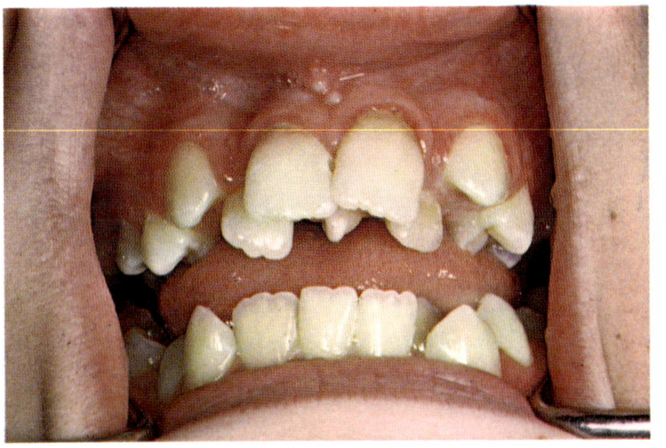

66

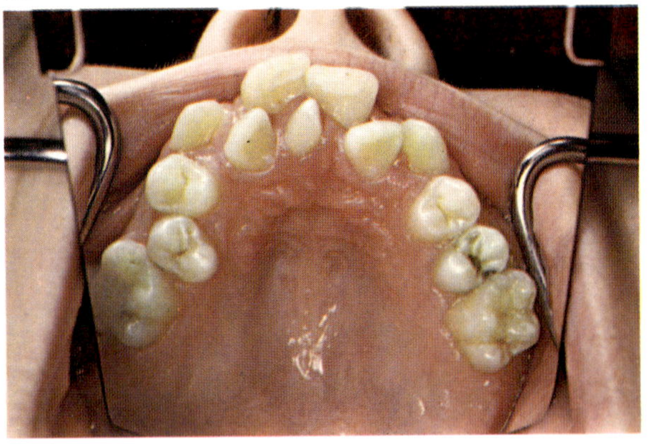

67 Mesiodens Conical mesiodens which has erupted into the line of the arch with premature loss of a primary incisor. Early removal will prevent disturbance of eruption of the permanent central incisor.

67

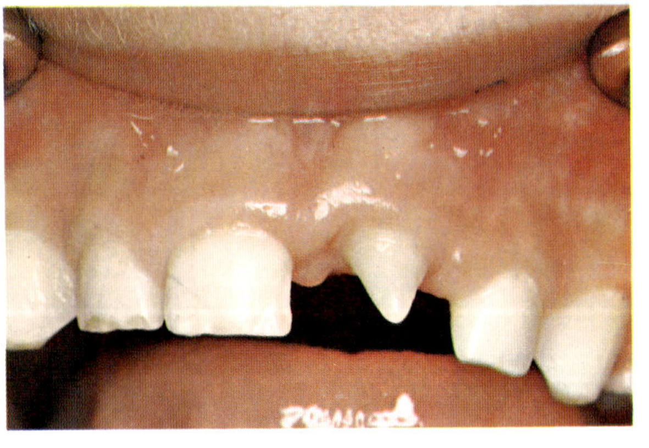

68 Mesiodens Inverted unilateral mesiodens seen in radiograph of maxillary incisor region lying between the apices of the central incisors. Caution must be exercised during the removal of this tooth to avoid injuring the neural and vascular supply of the incisor teeth.

68

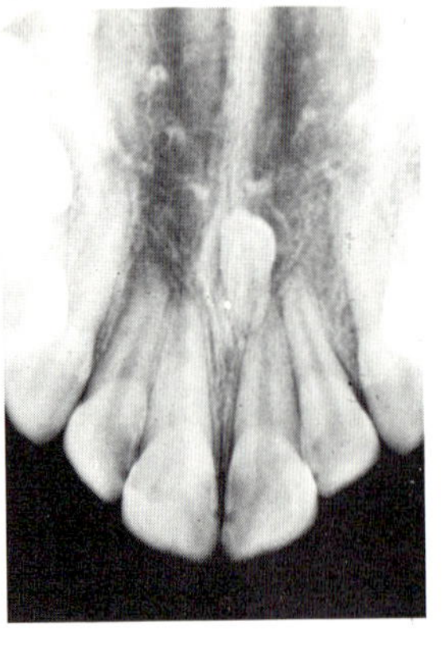

69 Retained primary incisors Retained maxillary primary central incisors in a 10 year old boy with erupted permanent lateral incisors. A frequent cause for this condition is the presence of mesiodentes.

69

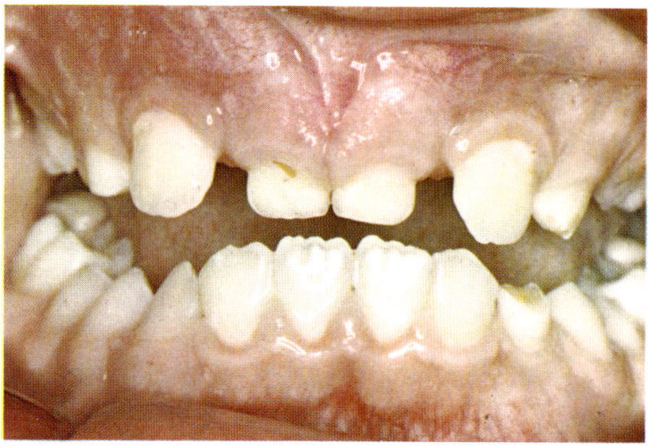

70 Bilateral mesiodens Bilateral tuberculate mesiodens shown in a radiograph of the premaxillary region seen in **69**. Note the considerable displacement and rotation of the permanent central incisors.

70

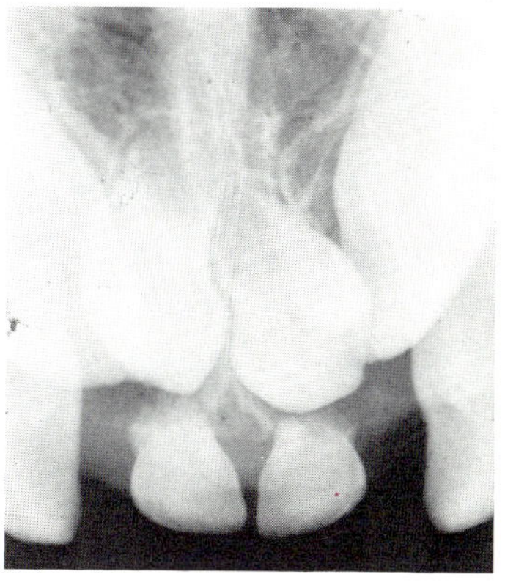

71 Supplemental permanent incisor Supplemental maxillary permanent lateral incisor. Comparison with the mesiodistal width of the lateral incisor in the adjacent quadrant may help to decide on the normal tooth.

71

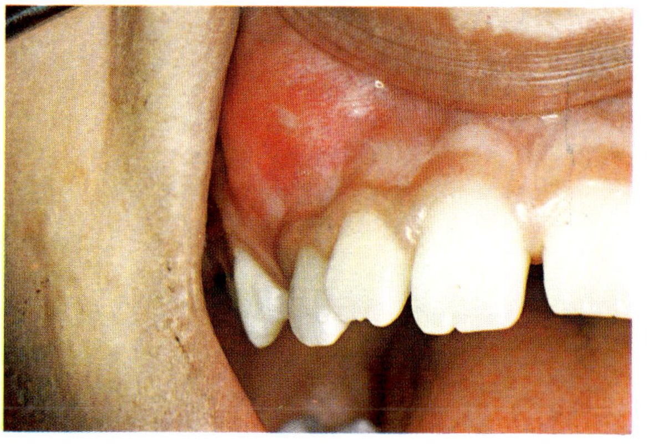

72 Root resorption Root resorption of the maxillary left central incisor associated with a mesiodens. The periapical radiograph was taken after trauma to the upper incisor teeth.

72

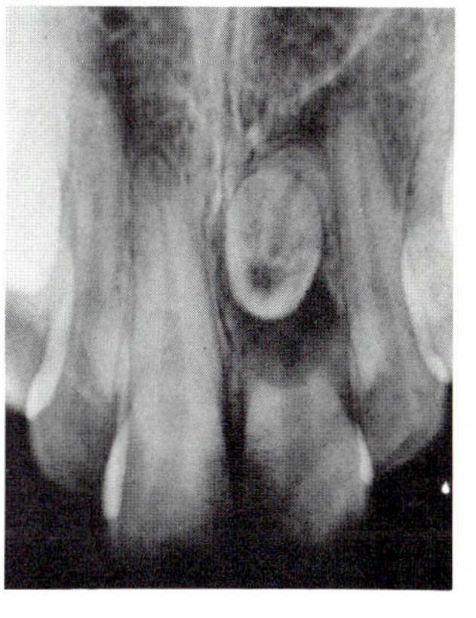

73 Supplemental permanent canine This rare supernumerary tooth is almost identical to the mesially placed normal canine. Retention of such teeth is dependent on the amount of space in the arch and the occlusion.

73

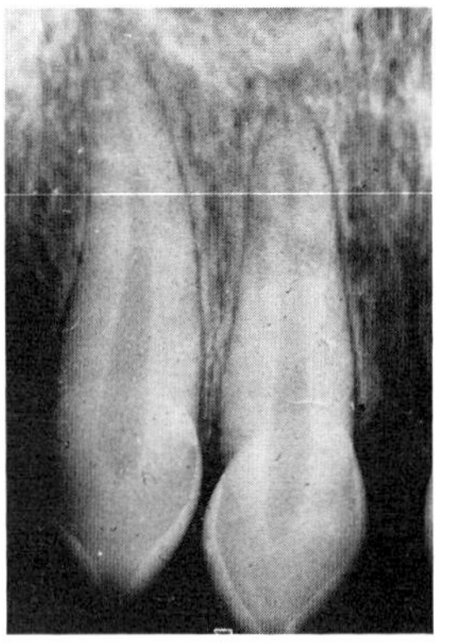

74 Supernumerary permanent canine Supernumerary permanent canine seen in a radiographic survey of the maxillary labial segment in the region of the right canine apex.

74

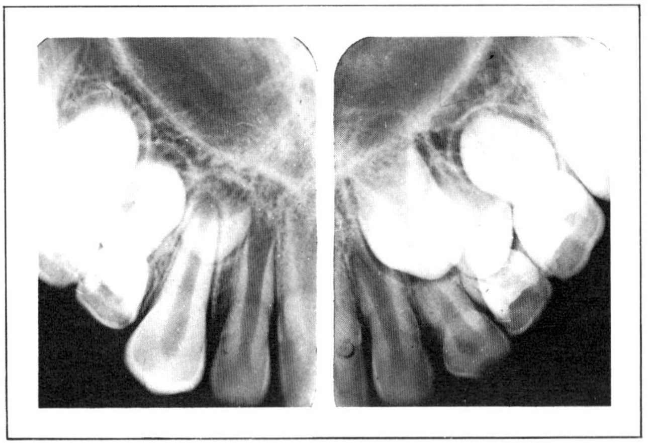

75 Bilateral supplemental mandibular premolars Additional premolars are more commonly seen in the mandible and are usually supplemental in form. Radiographs of this unusual case show two supplemental premolars on the right and one on the left.

75

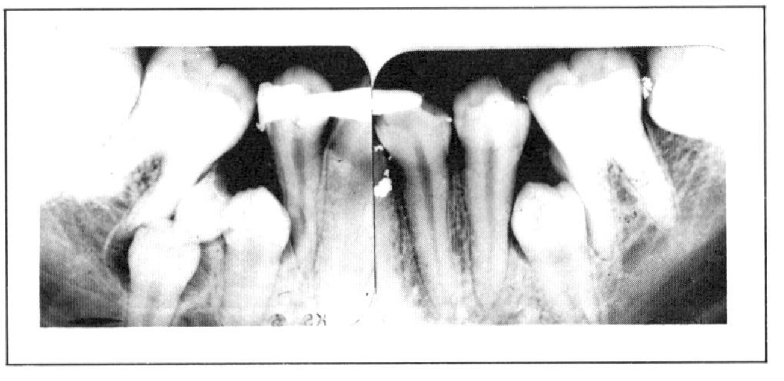

76 Bilateral supernumerary permanent molars (distomolars) As seen on the left side of the jaw in this radiograph, a supernumerary molar may impede the eruption of the third molar. Supernumerary teeth in the molar region are more common in the maxilla than in the mandible.

76

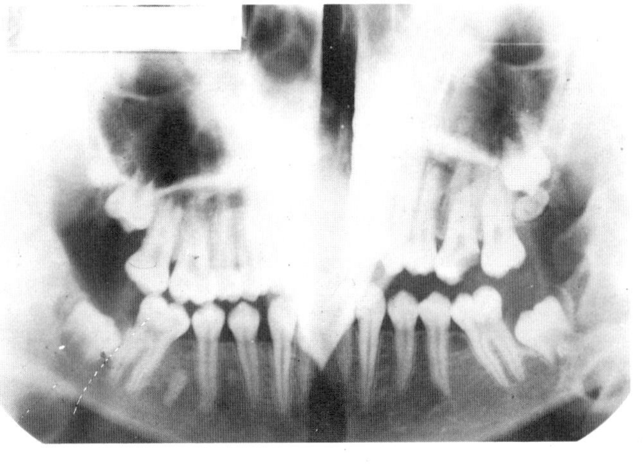

77 Supernumerary permanent molar An unusual tuberculate supernumerary impeding the eruption of the mandibular second molar.

77

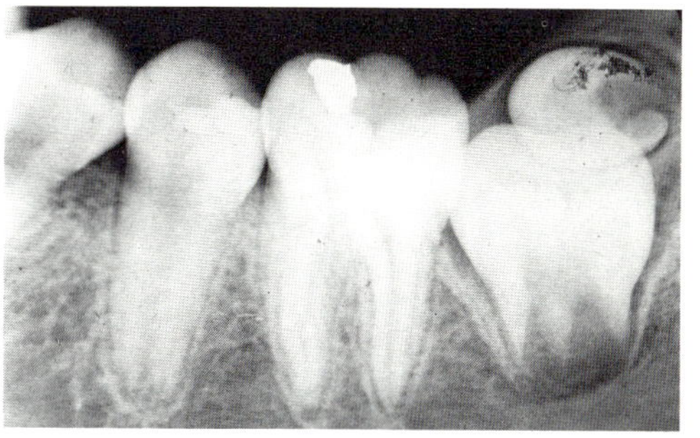

78 Supernumerary permanent molar Photograph of the tuberculate supernumerary seen in **77** after surgical removal.

78

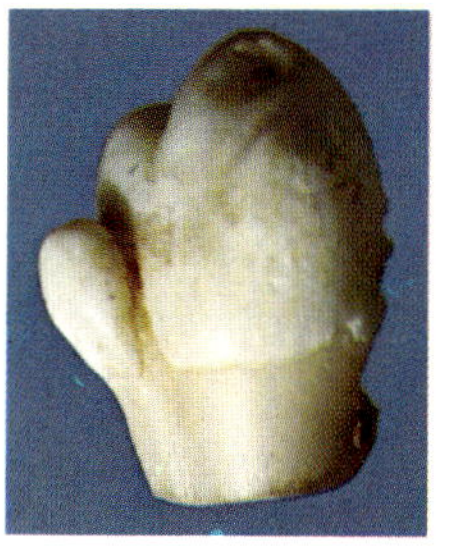

79 Cleidocranial dysostosis Radiographs of labial segments of the dental arches showing failure of eruption of many permanent incisor teeth and retention of the primary predecessors in 10 year old boy with cleidocranial dysostosis. Note the presence of many supernumerary teeth which are a major feature of this condition. (See **8**, **9** and **10**)

79

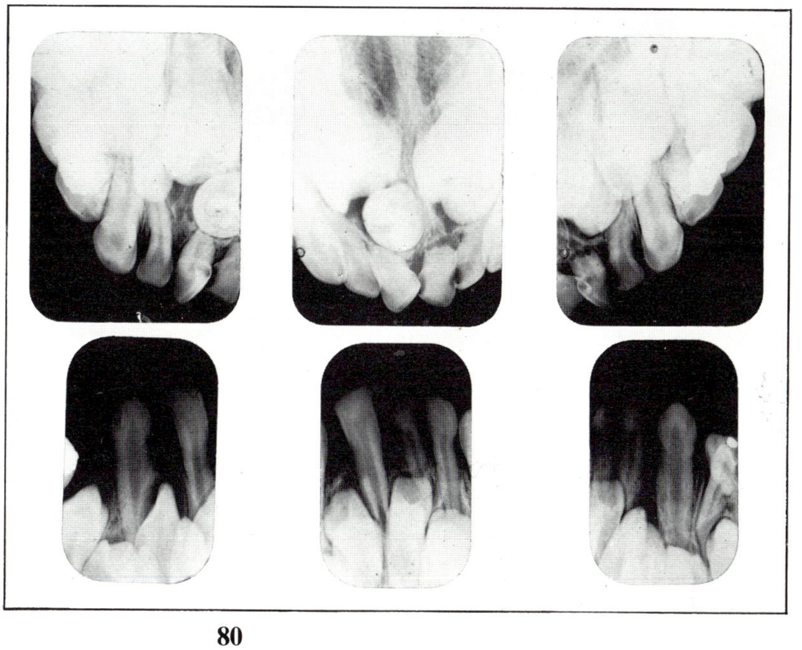

80 Supernumerary (Accessory) cusps Bilateral maxillary permanent central incisors with a supernumerary cusp arising from the palatal cingulum.

80

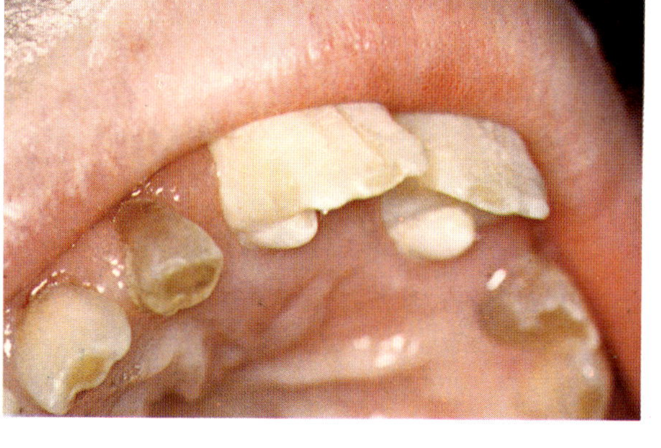

81 **Supernumerary (Accessory) cusp** Radiograph of maxillary central incisor showing well defined palatally placed supernumerary cusp. Note the prolongation of the pulpal shadow into the cusp. These large additional elements often interfere with the occlusion and require removal.

81

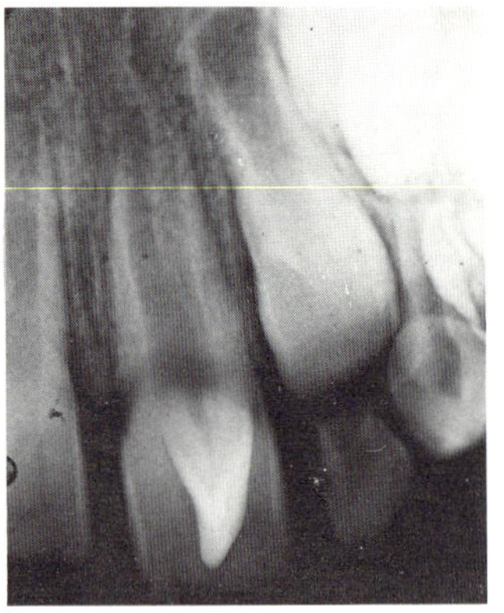

82 **Supernumerary (Accessory) cusp** Maxillary first primary molar with additional buccal cusp. In this instance it is seen in a case of incontinentia pigmenti (Bloch-Sulzberger syndrome) in which it is associated with severe hypodontia and other anomalies of dental morphology in the primary and permanent dentitions.

82

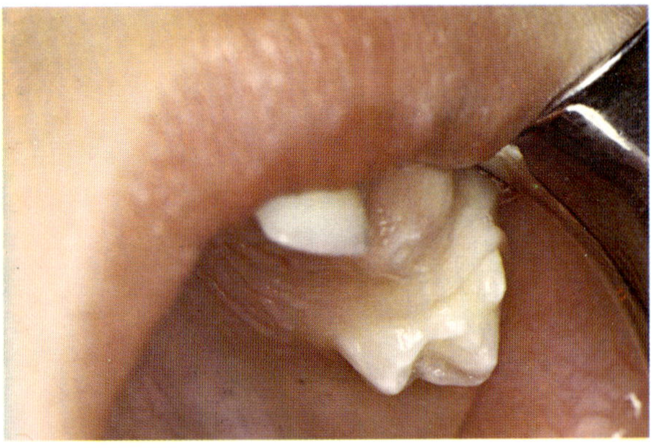

83 **Supernumerary (Accessory) cusp** Maxillary second molar with additional buccal element. The siting of these supernumerary cusps may predispose to caries or periodontal disease.

83

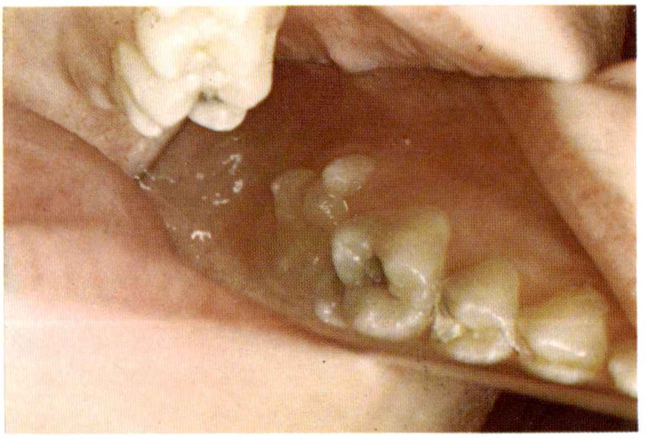

(ii) Hypodontia

84 **Avulsion** The maxillary permanent central incisor was avulsed at the age of 9 years. Subsequent mesial drift of the lateral incisor has almost closed the space. This case illustrates the necessity for an adequate history prior to the diagnosis of hypodontia and the need for a space maintainer.

84

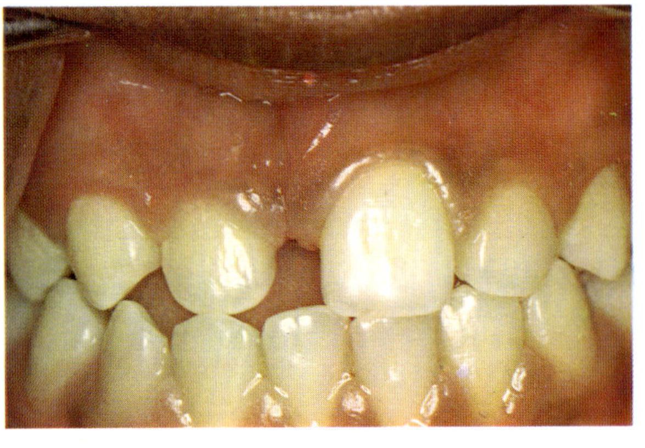

85 Hypodontia In this unusual case, the radiograph shows that the congenital absence of maxillary primary lateral incisors is associated with the absence of permanent successors.

85

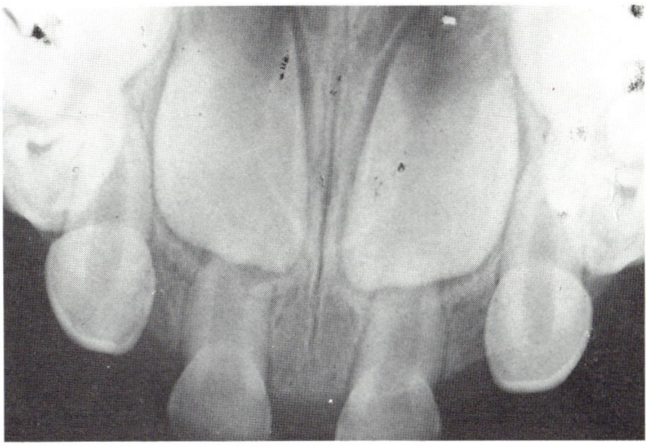

86 Hypodontia Congenital absence of a mandibular second premolar. Infraocclusion (submergence) of the primary molar may or may not be associated with hypodontias of this type. Excluding the third permanent molar, this is the most commonly missing tooth in Caucasian populations.

86

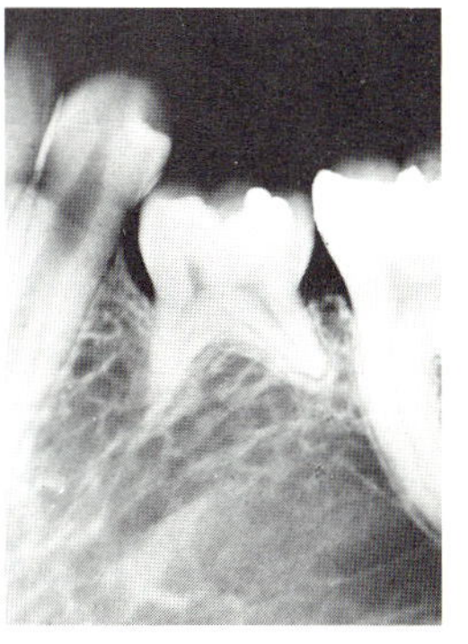

87 Hypodontia Bilateral congenital absence of maxillary lateral incisors associated, in this case, with the absence of a lower incisor in the permanent dentition.

87

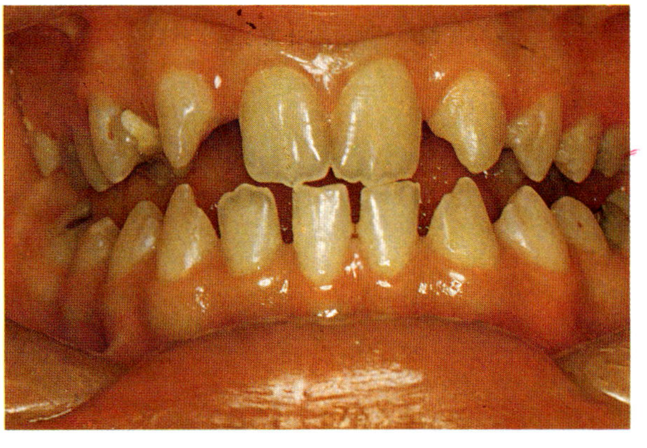

88 Hypodontia A radiograph taken to explain the prolonged retention of a primary mandibular incisor shows the congenital absence of the permanent successor. The rate of primary root resorption in cases of this type is extremely variable.

88

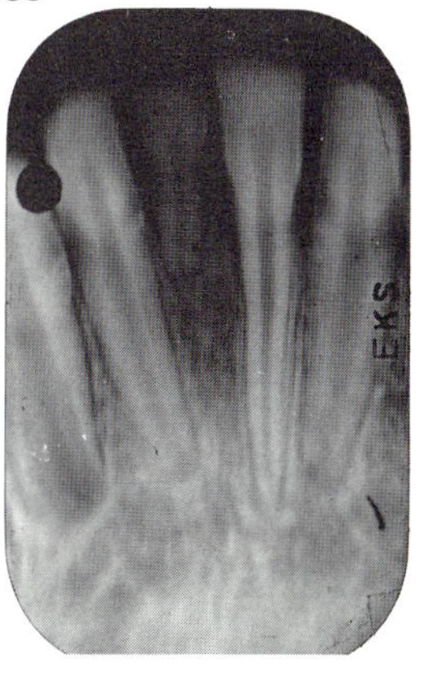

89

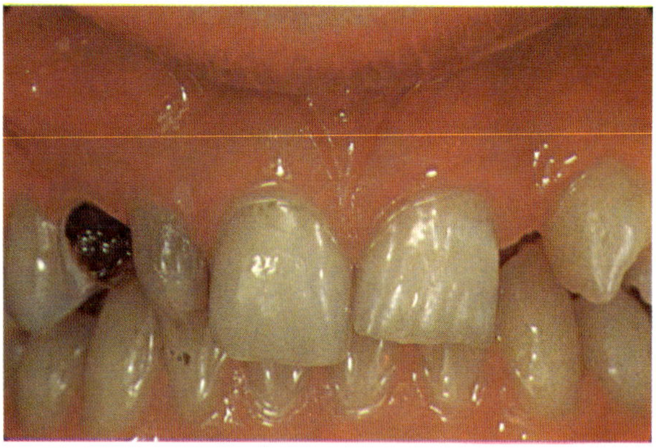

89 Hypodontia Congenital absence of maxillary left permanent lateral incisor associated with the presence of a conical 'peg-shaped' right lateral incisor. This association is occasionally seen in some members of families with bilateral congenital absence of maxillary lateral incisors.

90

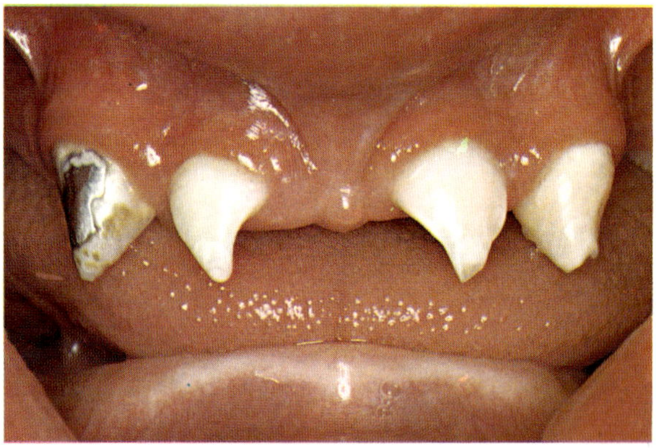

90 Hypodontia Severe hypodontia in the primary and permanent dentitions in this case is associated with X-linked recessive hypohidrotic ectodermal dysplasia. Note the total absence of teeth in the mandible and the characteristic conical deformity of the newly erupting maxillary permanent central incisors.

91

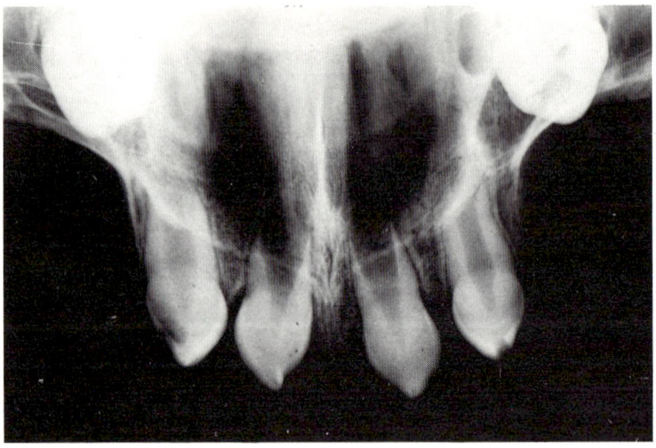

91 Radiograph of the case shown in **90**.

92

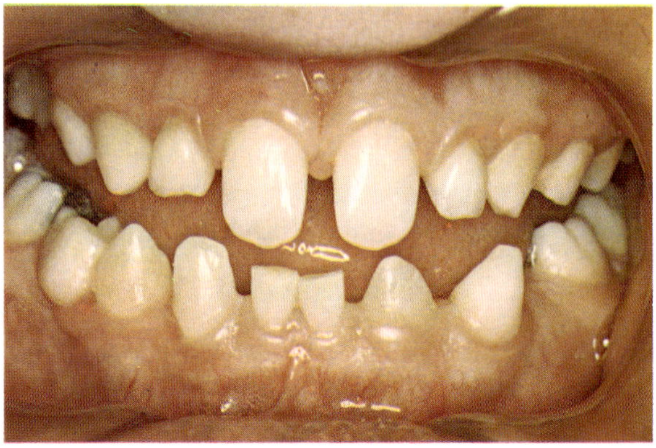

92 Hypodontia Severe hypodontia in the permanent dentition in this girl is associated with an autosomal dominant ectodermal dysplasia. Note the tapering coronal morphology of the maxillary permanent central incisors and the right mandibular permanent incisor.

93

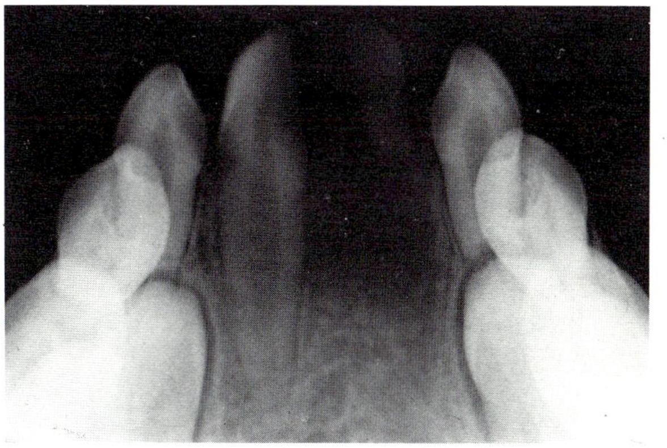

93 Hypodontia Radiograph of the mandibular incisor region showing congenital absence of both primary and permanent incisors in a 9 year old boy with Rieger's syndrome – a rare autosomal dominantly determined abnormality.

94

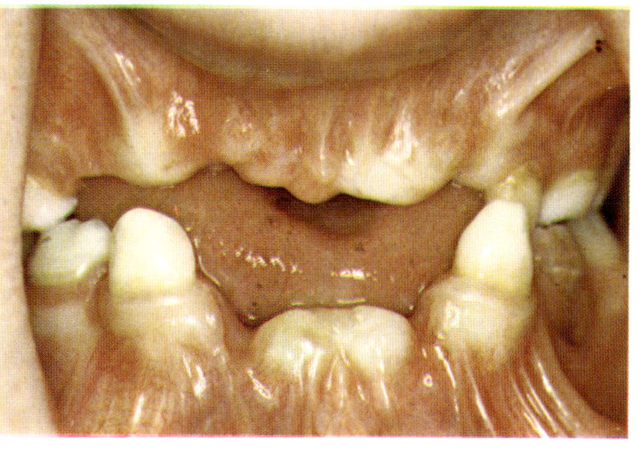

94 Hypodontia Congenital absence of primary and permanent teeth is especially marked in the incisor region in this case of chondroectodermal dysplasia (Ellis-van Creveld syndrome). Note the characteristic fusion of lip mucosa to gingiva with obliteration of the labial sulci in upper and lower jaws in this 4 year old boy.

95

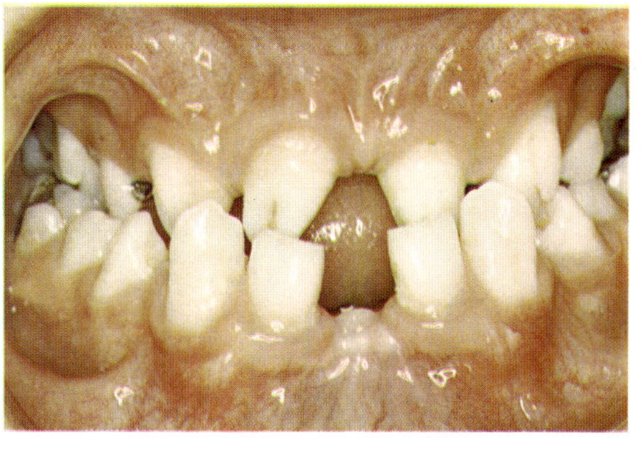

95 Hypodontia The congenital absence of teeth in this 17 year old boy with chondroectodermal dysplasia (Ellis-van Creveld syndrome) is less marked than in the previous case. Hypodontia is most evident in the incisor region with absence of the mandibular primary central incisors and all mandibular permanent incisors as well as the maxillary lateral incisors. Note the conical deformity of the maxillary central incisors and the multiple frena tethering the upper lip mucosa to the gingiva.

b. Shape of primary and permanent teeth

(i) External

96 Double primary tooth (Fusion) This anomaly is probably due to fusion of the mandibular lateral incisor and canine. It is frequently associated with abnormalities in the underlying permanent dentition, such as missing or supernumerary teeth.

96

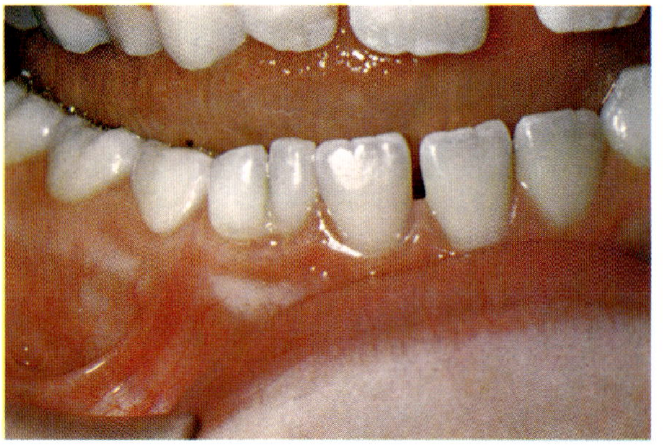

97

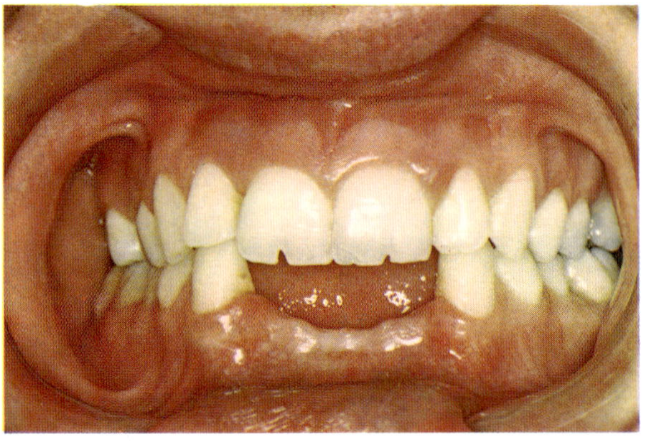

97 Double permanent tooth (Gemination) The large mesio-distal diameter of the crowns and notching of the incisal edges of these maxillary permanent central incisors show evidence of possible partial gemination of the tooth germs. A radiograph (**125**) confirms the presence of double coronal pulp chambers and single root canal.

98

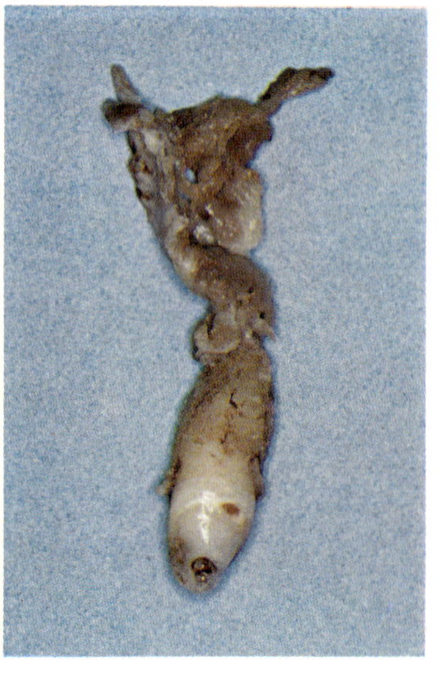

98 Dens invaginatus (Dens in dente) The conical deformity of the crown of this invaginated maxillary lateral incisor is typical of the more severe varieties of dens invaginatus (dens in dente). This tooth was surgically removed together with an associated apical cyst. Infection of the pulp via the enamel invagination and subsequent pulpal necrosis is a frequent complication of these anomalies.

99 Dilaceration The distortion of the partially erupted maxillary left permanent central incisor is due to a dilaceration injury produced by trauma to the primary predecessor.

99

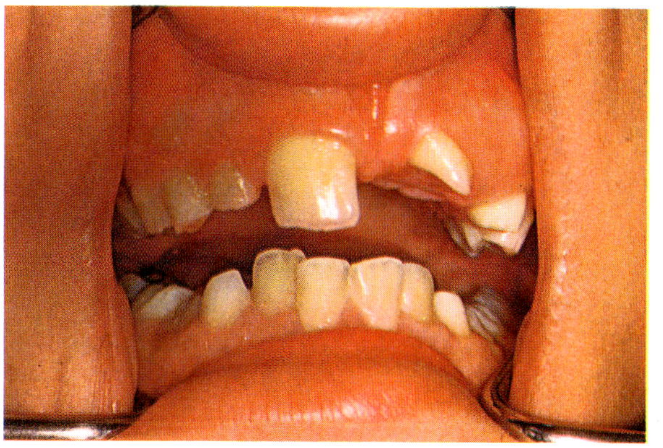

100 Dilaceration Trauma to the mandibular primary incisors during early childhood resulted in injury to the underlying permanent right central incisor crown. This radiograph shows the dilaceration injury at the crown/root junction. The tooth remained vital.

100

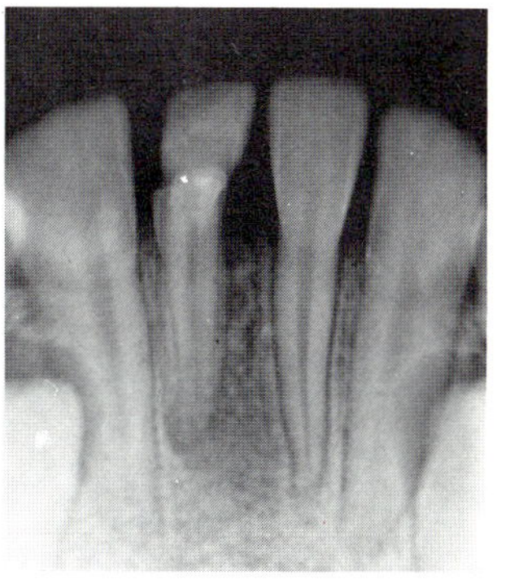

101 Dilaceration Radiograph of a dilacerated maxillary central incisor caused by early trauma to the primary predecessor. Avulsion and intrusion of a primary incisor are the types of injury likely to lead to this kind of deformity.

102 Dilaceration Lateral view of surgically removed dilacerated incisor seen in **101**. The dilaceration has occurred at the crown/root junction. These severe deformities are inconsistent with normal eruption and require surgical removal.

101

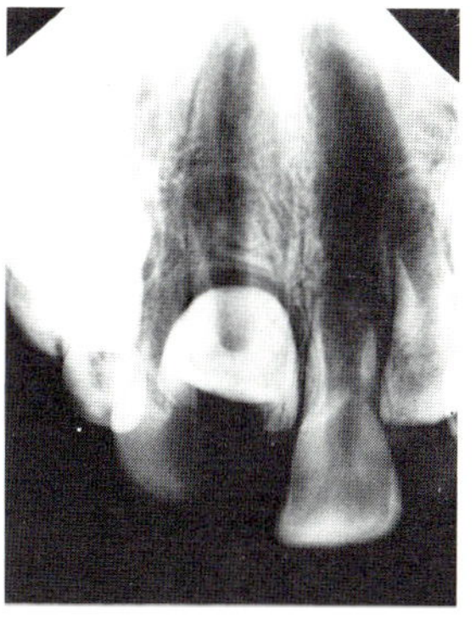

102

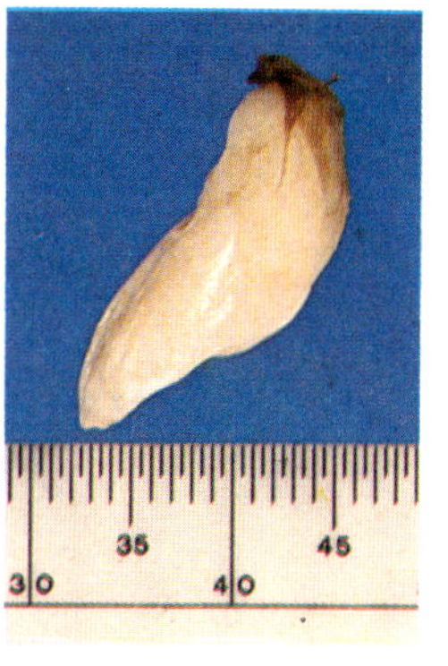

103 Hutchinson's incisor Abnormal tooth form is one of the stigmata of congenital syphilis. This case demonstrates the typical barrel-shaped incisor morphology in both jaws.

103

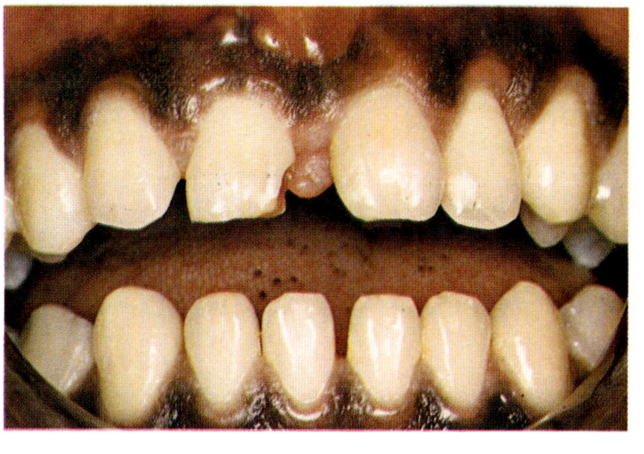

104 Moon's molar The severe disturbance of coronal morphology of the first permanent molar is another characteristic of congenital syphilis.

104

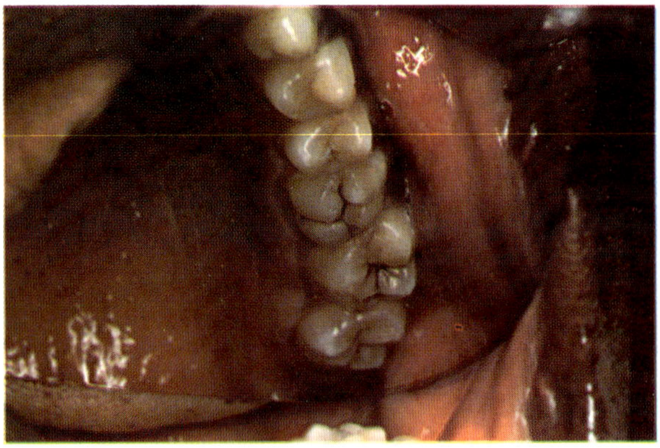

105 Mulberry molar Hypoplasia of the early mineralising portions of the first permanent molar crown is occasionally associated with congenital syphilis and is described as a 'mulberry' molar.

105

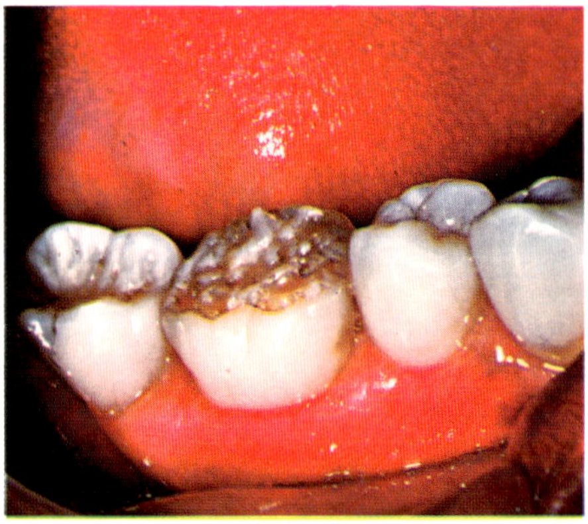

106 Conical incisors The crowns of two mandibular permanent central incisors are conical in shape. There is no evidence of associated hypodontia.

106

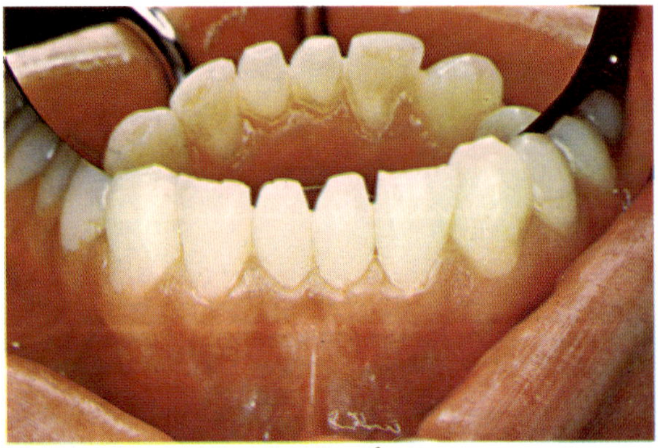

107 Conical incisors Maxillary central incisor teeth in both the primary and permanent dentitions are seen to have a conical coronal form. Congenital absence of lateral incisors in both dentitions is also evident. These anomalies were, however, confined to the dentition and no evidence of more generalised forms of ectodermal dysplasia could be seen.

107

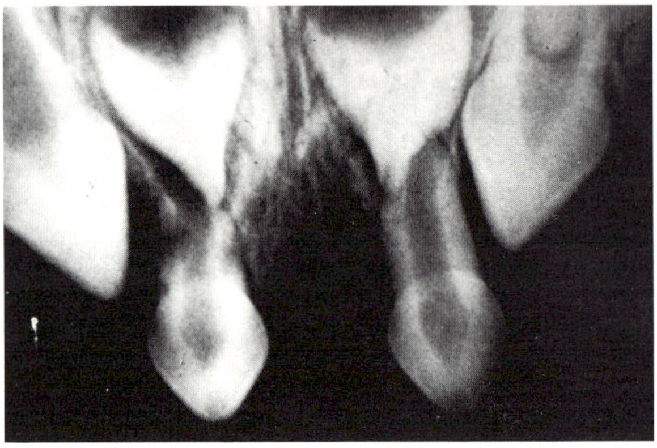

108 Erosion Enamel loss from the labial aspects of these maxillary primary incisors was caused by the erosive effect of excessive fruit juice consumption from a feeding bottle in infancy.

108

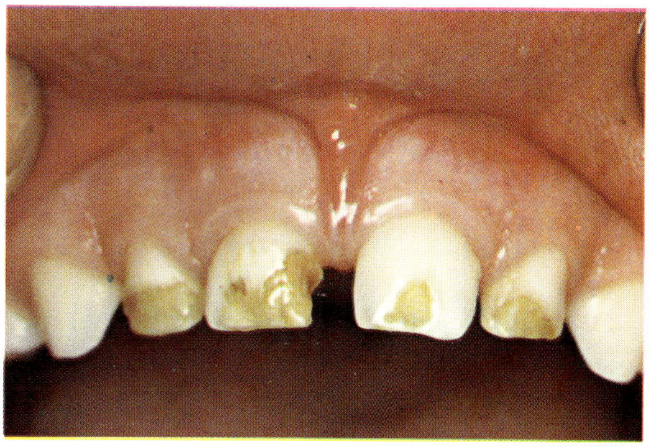

109 Attrition Physiological wear on primary teeth during mastication is common in young children. This process may be accelerated in some individuals who are in the habit of nocturnal grinding. Mentally retarded or cerebral palsied children may be subject to severe grinding movements throughout the day and night, with resultant gross attrition. Dentine frequently becomes exposed by such activity.

109

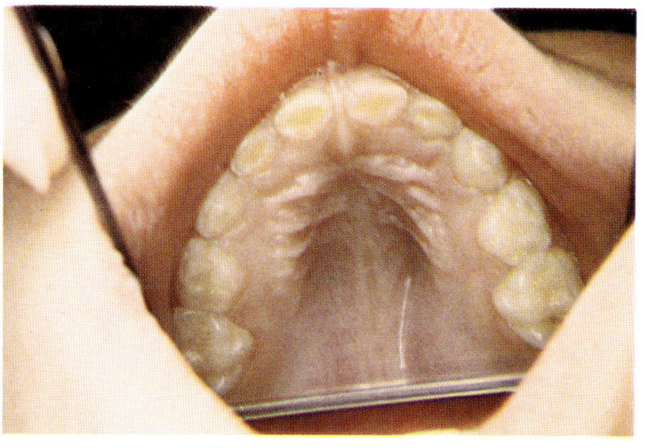

110, 111 Globodontia The curious globular deformity of the crowns of premolar and molar teeth seen in the upper and lower jaws of this case is typical of the otodental syndrome. These individuals are subject to high frequency deafness from childhood. The other dental anomalies associated with this syndrome are fusion of molar and premolar teeth and double pulp chambers in these teeth.

110

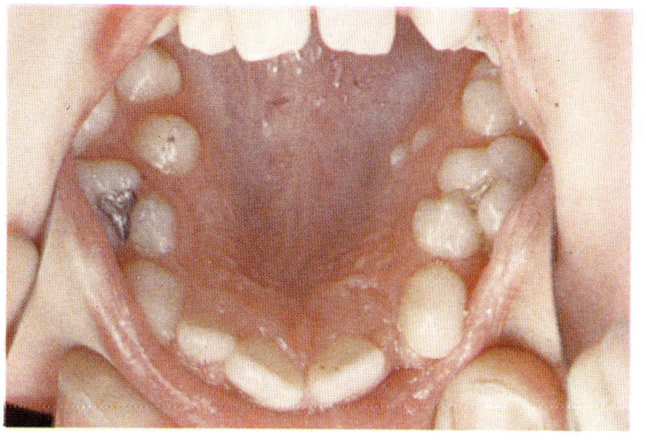

111

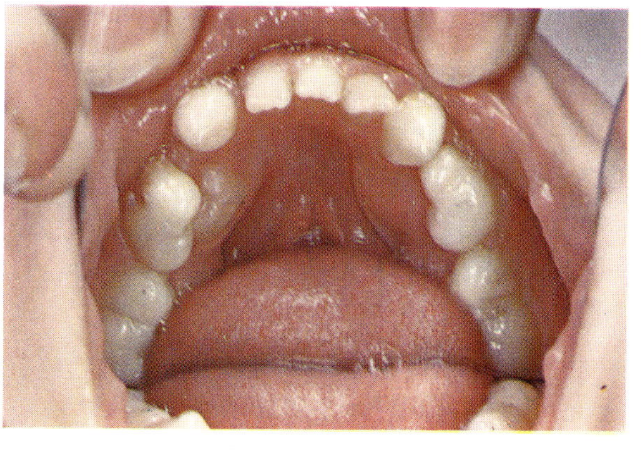

112 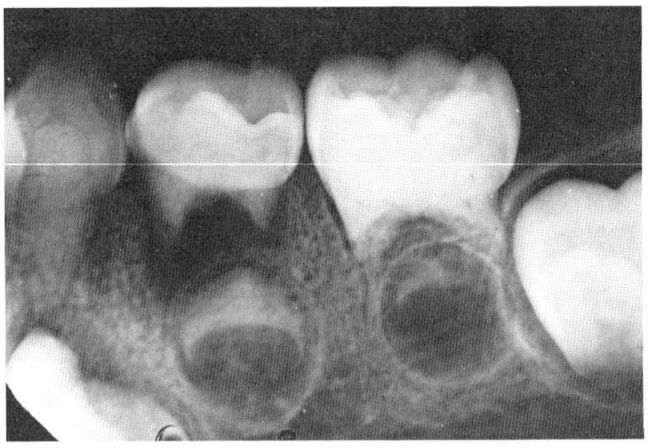

112 Dentinogenesis imperfecta (Hereditary opalescent dentine) The bulbous crowns, short spiky roots and total calcific obliteration of the pulp spaces of the primary teeth are all characteristic of this anomaly. The periapical and inter-radicular rarefaction seen affecting the first primary molar despite the pulpal calcification is also a feature of this condition.

113 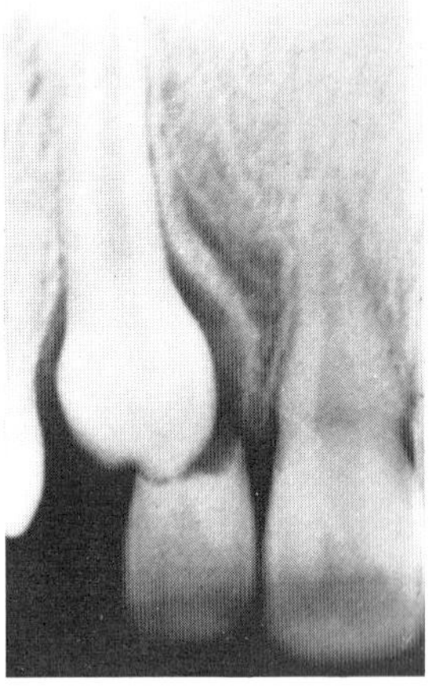

113 Root resorption The root of a permanent lateral incisor may occasionally be resorbed by pressure from an ectopically erupting permanent canine.

114 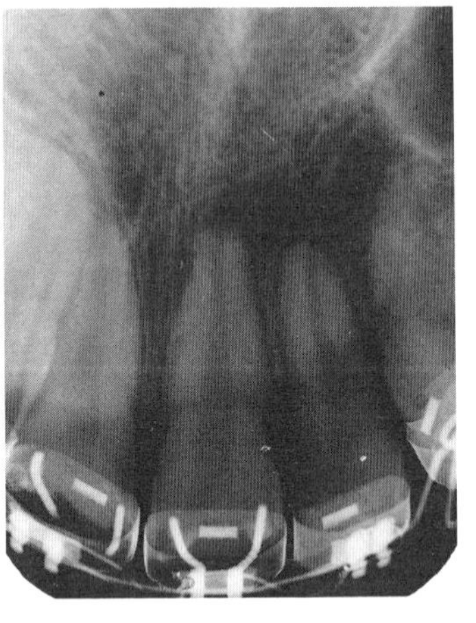

114 Root resorption The apices of the maxillary permanent central and lateral incisor are undergoing root resorption which is associated with rapid orthodontic tooth movement.

(ii) Internal

115 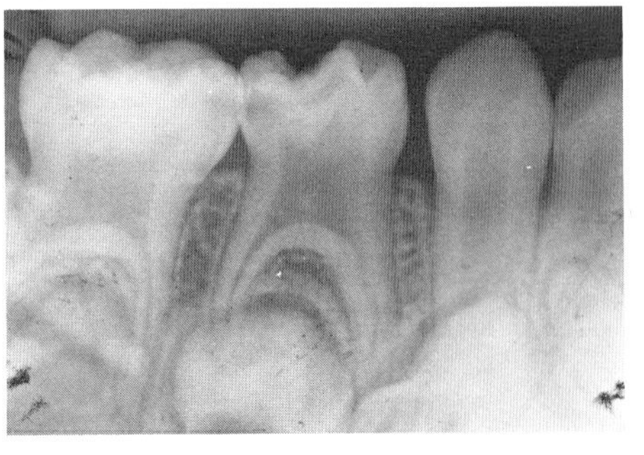

115 Taurodontism The mandibular first and second primary molars manifest enlarged pulp chambers through apparent apical extension of the trunks of the teeth. The roots are correspondingly short. Although this child is otherwise normal, similar findings have been noted in hypohidrotic ectodermal dysplasia and Klinefelter's syndrome.

116 Dens invaginatus Radiograph showing the typical pear-shaped enamel invagination extending from the palatal cingulum superimposed on the pulpal shadow of the maxillary lateral incisor.

116

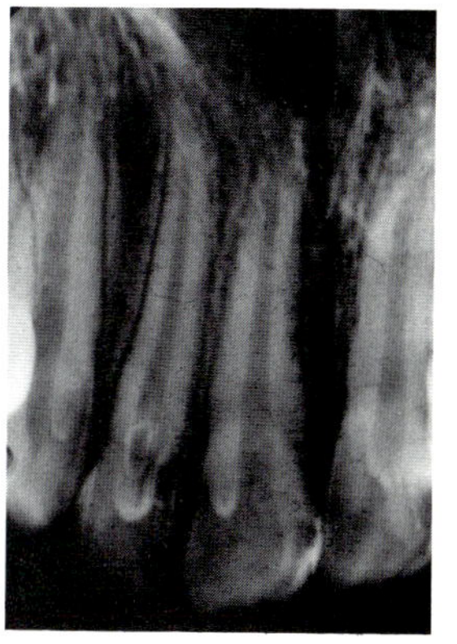

117 Dens invaginatus The large area of disto-apical bony rarefaction associated with the invaginated and non-vital maxillary left lateral incisor was observed in routine radiographic examination of this 15 year old girl. The lesion resolved completely after endodontic treatment and root filling. Prophylactic restoration of both invaginated lateral incisors had been undertaken at the same age, the right lateral incisor remaining vital.

117

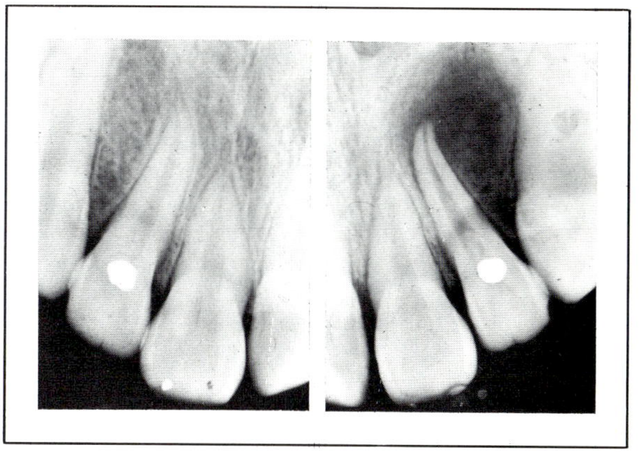

118 Dens invaginatus (Dens in dente) This radiograph shows the appearance of one of the more severe forms of coronal enamel invagination affecting the maxillary lateral incisor. The appearance of this variety led to the use of the term 'dens in dente'. It is characterised by a conical coronal form, with the orifice of the invagination near to the incisal tip and a grossly dilated root form. These anomalies almost invariably become infected and as seen in this case, are commonly associated with periapical bony rarefaction.

118

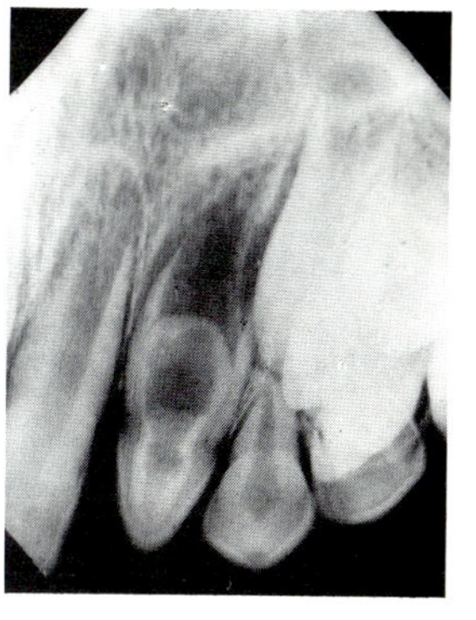

119 Dens invaginatus (Dens in dente) The maxillary lateral incisor is affected by two invaginations. One of these may be seen on the mesial aspect of the root.

120 Dens invaginatus (Dens in dente) The enamel lined root invagination described in **119** is clearly seen in this photograph of the tooth after surgical removal.

119

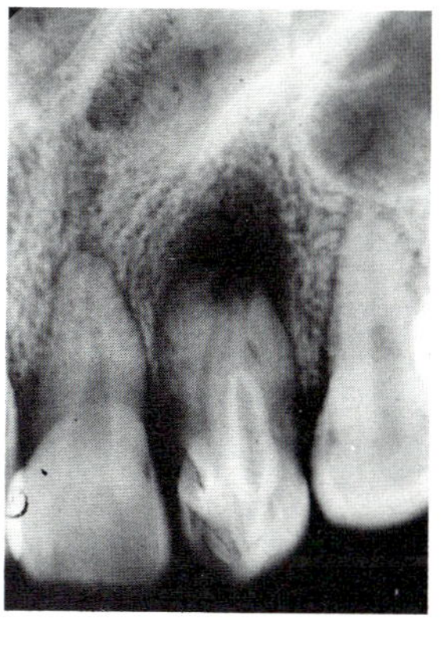

120

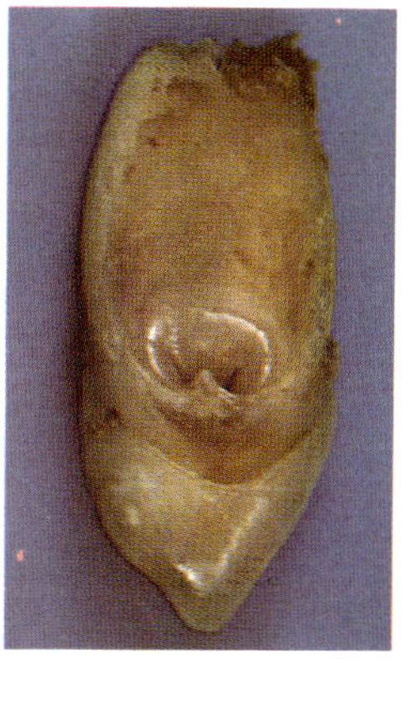

121 Dens evaginatus (Tuberculated premolar) The mandibular left second premolar in this 12 year old Indian boy shows the presence of an occlusal tubercle in the central portion of the crown.

121

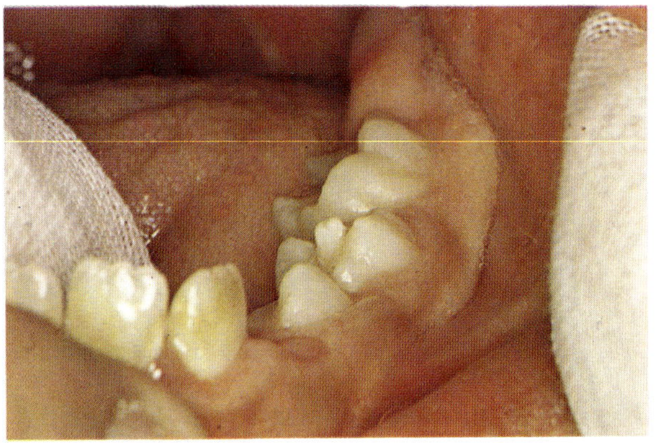

122 Radiograph of the affected tooth seen in **121** showing prolongation of the pulp space into the tubercle. Attrition of a similar tubercle on the antimere premolar resulted in pulpal exposure and acute dentoalveolar abscess formation. Anomalies of this type are common in individuals of Mongolian stock and may occur rarely in Caucasians.

122

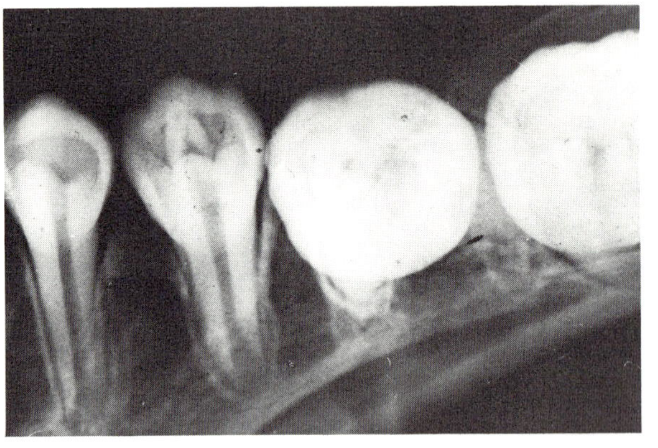

123 Double primary tooth (Fusion) Radiographic appearance of the fusion of two primary incisors with complete separation of the pulp chambers and root canals.

123

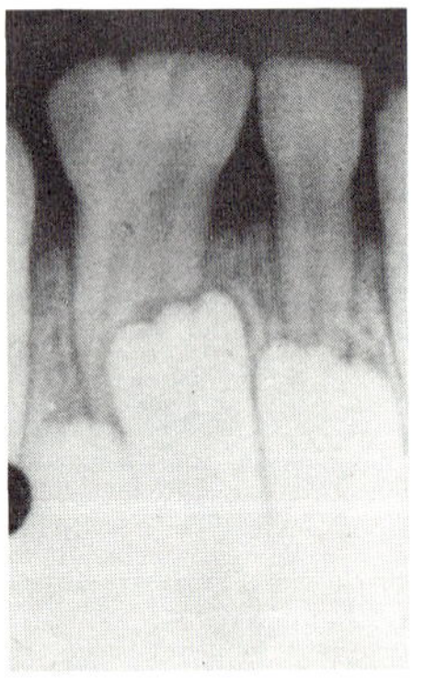

124 Double primary tooth (Gemination) In this double primary incisor, the pulp chambers appear to be separate but there is a common root canal. This form is probably caused by incomplete gemination of a tooth germ.

124

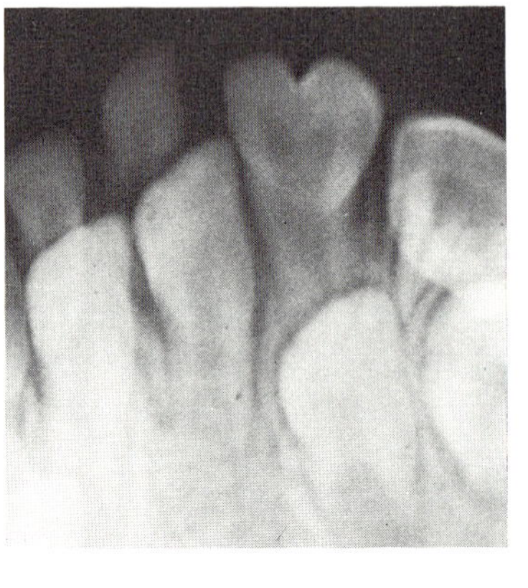

125

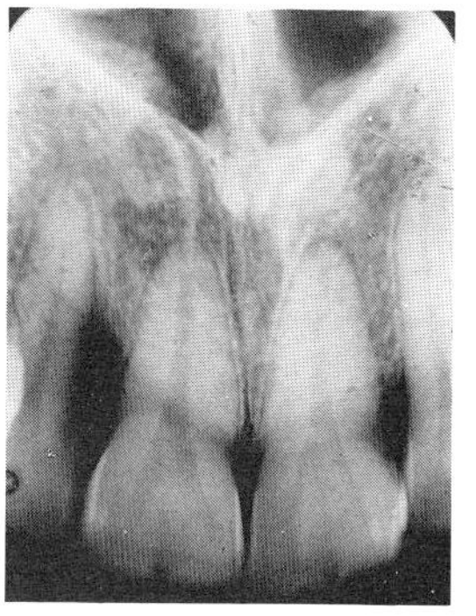

125 Double permanent tooth (Gemination) Radiographic appearance of the maxillary central incisors seen in **97** showing double pulp chambers and single root canals in each tooth. Incomplete gemination of the tooth germs may account for these anomalies.

126

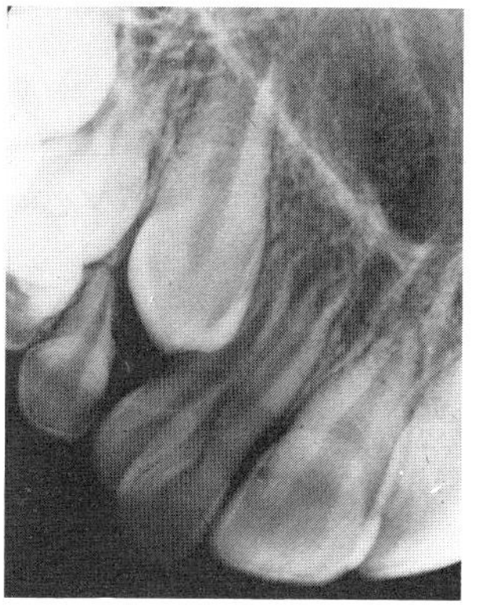

126 Double permanent tooth (Fusion) Radiograph of a double maxillary lateral incisor with separation of pulp chambers and root canals. This may be due to fusion of a normal tooth with a supernumerary element.

127

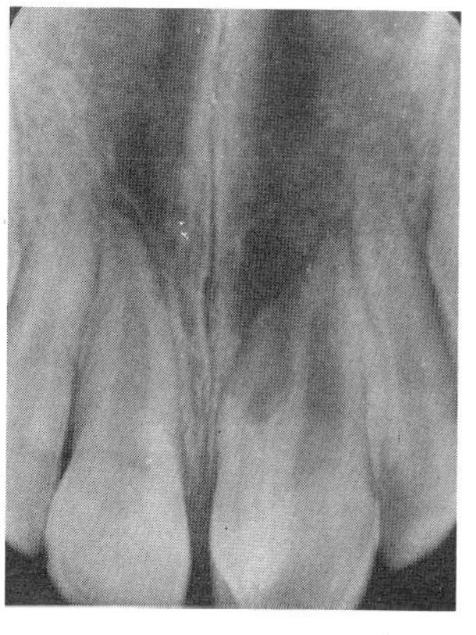

127 Double permanent tooth (Fusion) Radiograph of a maxillary permanent central incisor fused with a supernumerary element, showing evidence of two completely separate root canals.

128

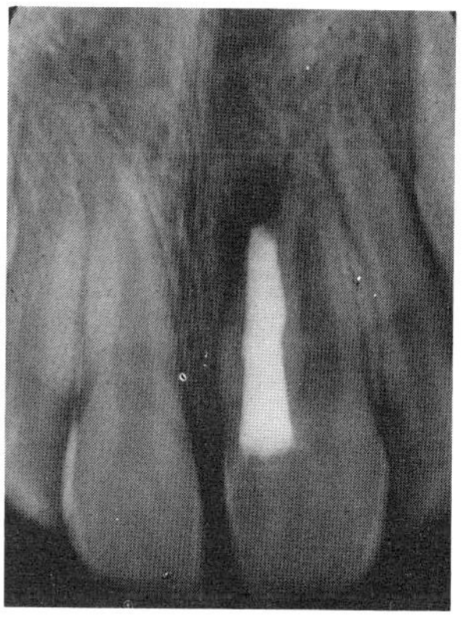

128 This second radiograph of the case seen in **127** shows the result of filling the root canal in the supernumerary element and of reshaping the crown into a more normal form.

129

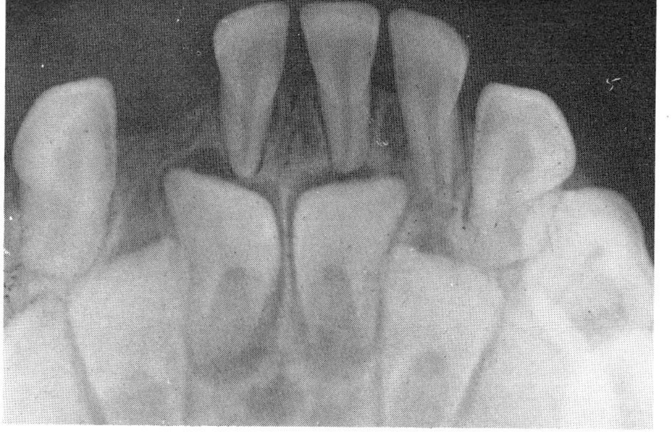

129 Hypodontia In this unusual case, the mandibular primary lateral incisor is congenitally absent and the parents were concerned about the possible absence of a permanent successor. The radiograph shows that the permanent lateral incisor is present.

130 Internal resorption A vital pulpotomy had been undertaken on this mandibular second primary molar 6 months previously, in which calcium hydroxide was utilised to dress the pulpal remnants at the entrance to the root canals. Marked internal resorption involving the upper portions of both root canals can be seen.

130

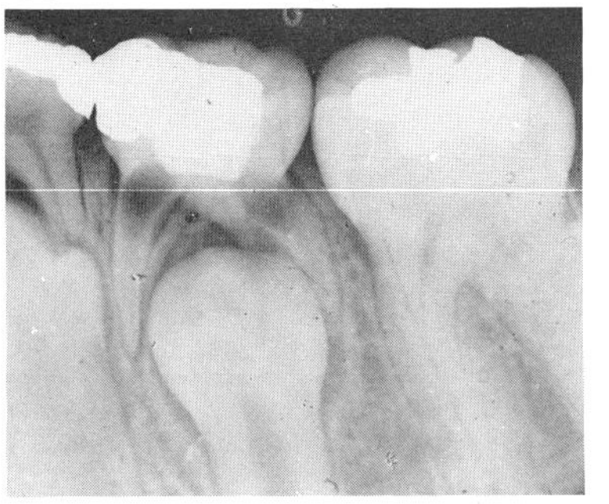

131 Internal resorption This radiograph shows evidence of internal resorption of the middle portions of the root canal of a heavily restored maxillary lateral incisor.

131

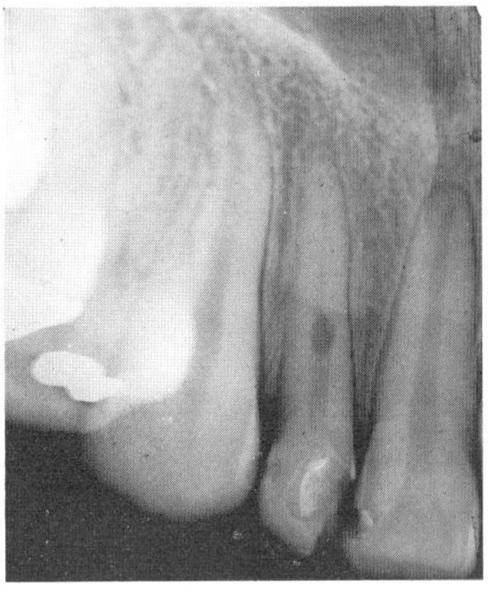

132 Calcific 'dentine' bridge Success for the calcium hydroxide type vital pulpotomy of cariously exposed primary molar pulps may be determined by the radiographic presence of a calcific bridge in the coronal portions of the root canals.

132

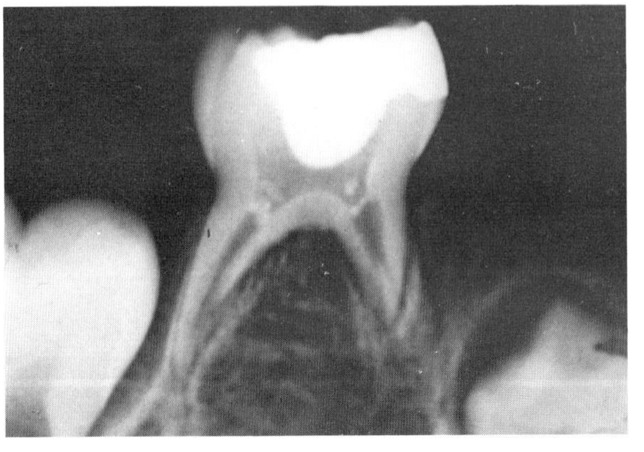

133 Dentine bridge This immature maxillary left permanent central incisor shows radiographic evidence of successful calcific bridging of the root canal beneath a calcium hydroxide dressing used in a vital pulpotomy procedure for a recent traumatic exposure.

133

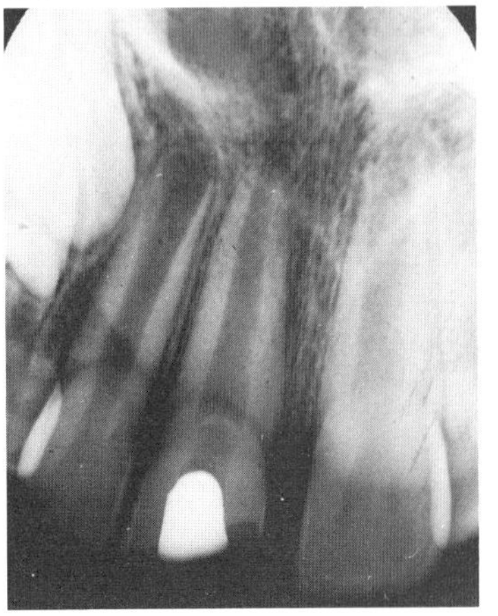

134 Pulpal calcification Dystrophic calcification of the pulp following trauma may lead to almost total obliteration of the pulp space, as seen in this radiograph of the maxillary right central incisor. A root fracture is also evident.

134

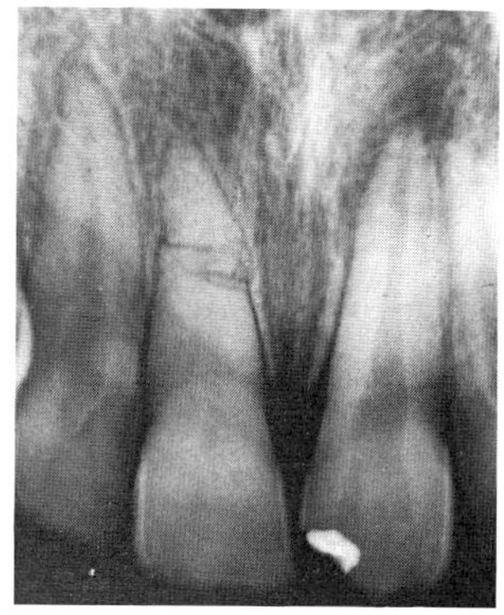

135 Dentinogenesis imperfecta (Hereditary opalescent dentine) Almost total calcific obliteration of the pulp spaces of both the primary incisors and the unerupted permanent incisor teeth may be seen. The bulbous crowns of the maxillary central incisors are another characteristic feature of this hereditary defect of dentine formation. Note the periapical area of rarefaction affecting the left primary central incisor.

135

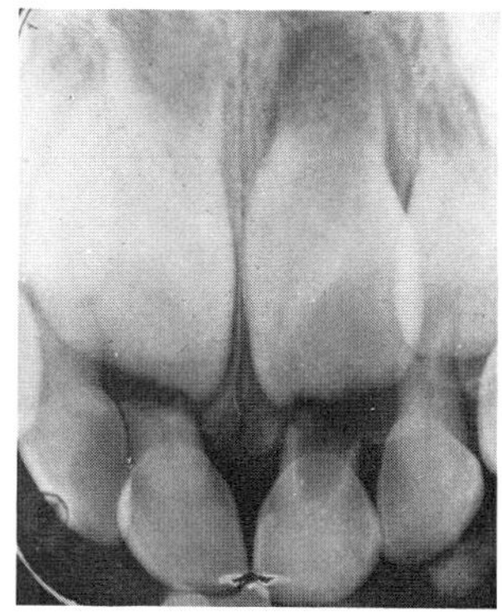

136 Dentinogenesis imperfecta (Hereditary opalescent dentine) The rapidity with which the pulp chambers of affected permanent incisor teeth are obliterated by abnormal dentine formation is illustrated in these radiographs, in which root formation is still incomplete. Note also the characteristic bulbous crowns.

136

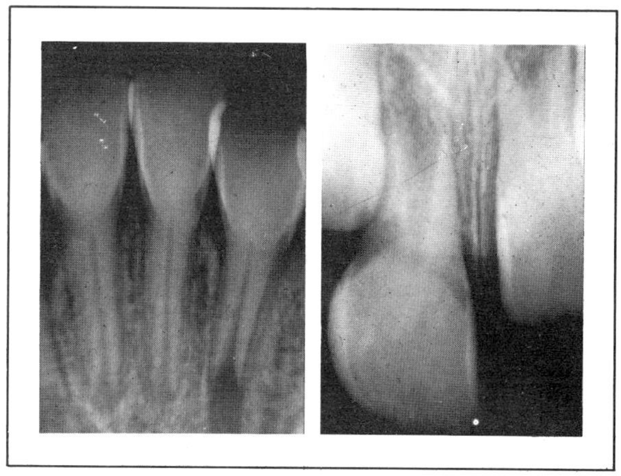

137 Coronal dentine dysplasia In this rare autosomal dominant defect the pulp canals are almost completely occluded by abnormal dentine formation, but a flame-shaped coronal pulp remains evident radiographically. As seen in the mandibular right central incisor, a portion of the flame-shaped pulp chamber may be occupied by a central pulp stone.

137

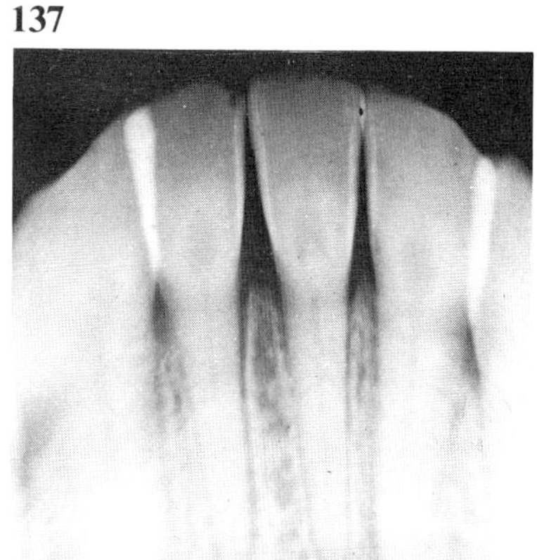

138 Multiple pulp stones These bitewing radiographs show evidence of multiple pulpal calcifications involving many of the premolar and molar teeth. The condition was asymptomatic.

138

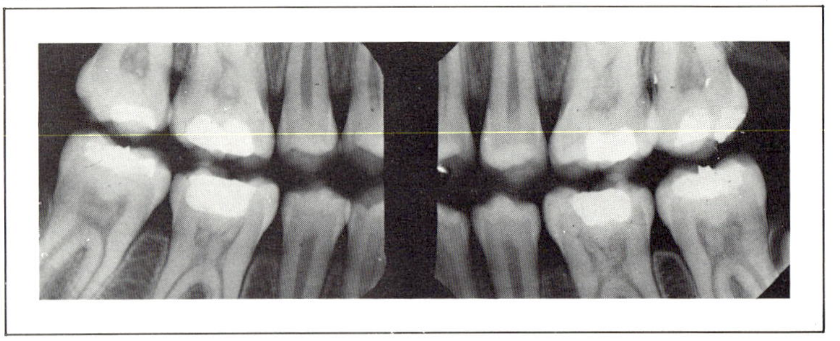

139 Pulp stone Section of a permanent incisor tooth showing a centrally placed pulpal calcification.

139

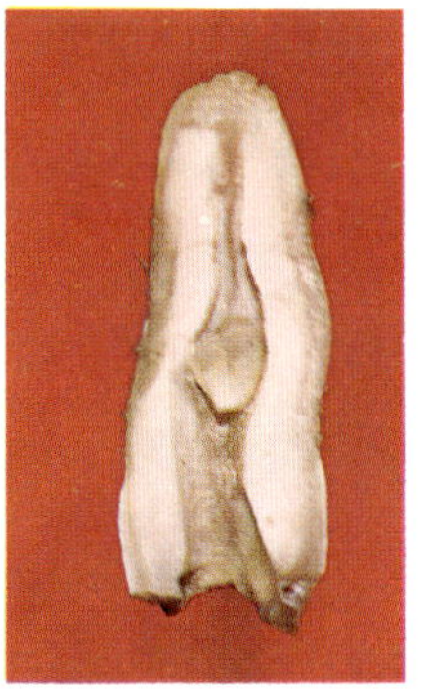

140 Hypophosphatasia The enlarged pulp spaces of these primary incisors and the periradicular bony rarefaction around the maxillary right central incisor, which is in the process of exfoliation, are two characteristic radiographic features seen in hypophosphatasia.

140

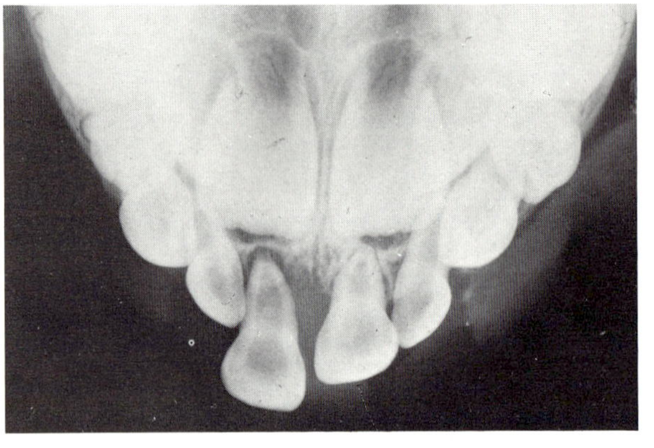

141, 142 Vitamin D resistant rickets (Hereditary hypophosphataemic rickets) The markedly enlarged mesial pulp horns of the second primary molars, the generally enlarged pulp spaces in the maxillary primary incisors and the pathological bony rarefaction around the maxillary right lateral incisor are all radiographic features seen in cases of X-linked dominant vitamin D resistant rickets. (See **177**, **178** and **478**)

141

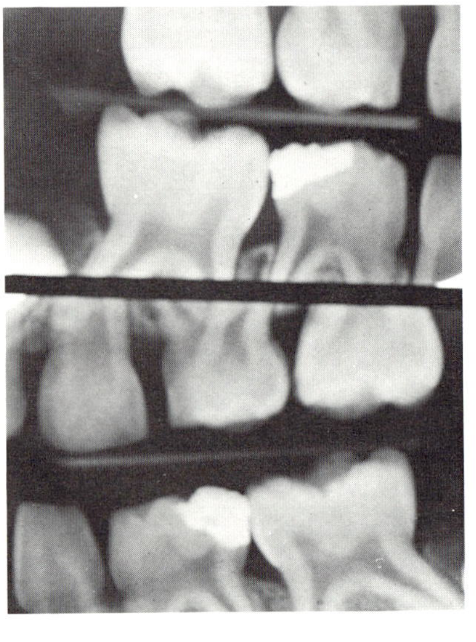

142

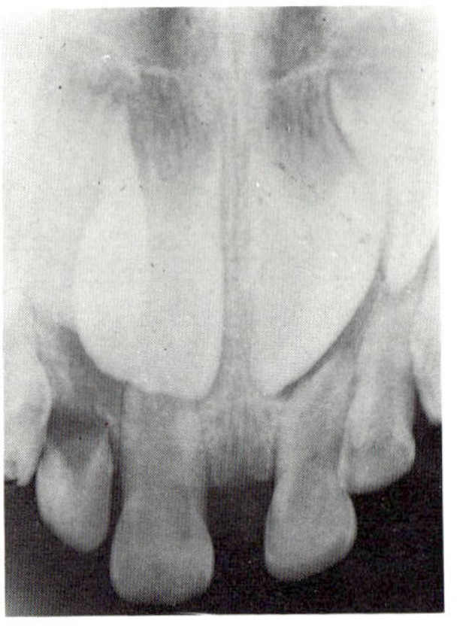

c. Size

143

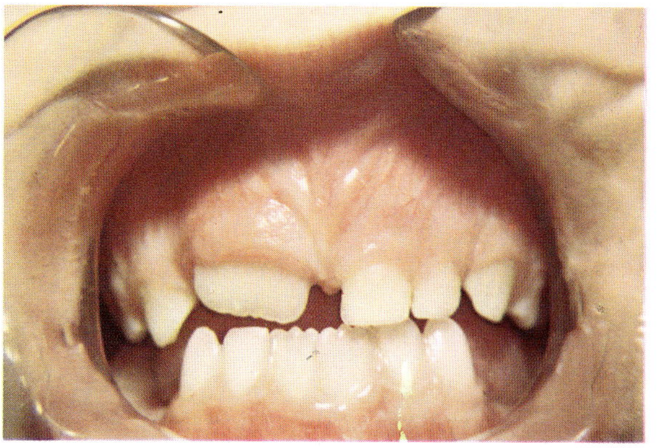

143 Macrodontia (Megadontia) The mesiodistal width of the erupted maxillary right permanent central incisor is well above the normal (80 per cent) range of 7.7–9.2mm. These grossly enlarged teeth invariably produce crowding in the arch and a marring of the facial appearance.

144

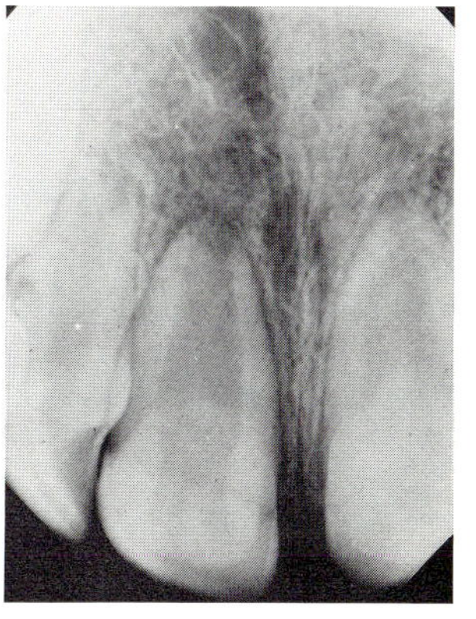

144 Macrodontia (Megadontia) This radiograph of a macrodont maxillary permanent central incisor shows evidence of a single pulp chamber and root canal; a feature distinguishing it from a double (geminated) tooth.

145

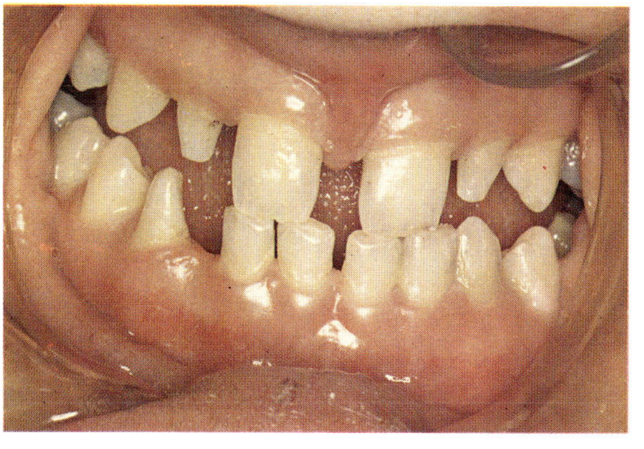

145 Microdontia All the permanent teeth are abnormally small with resultant spacing in the arches.

146

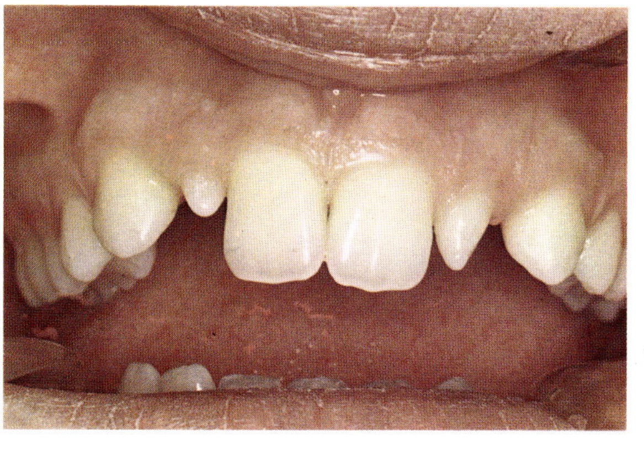

146 Microdontia The maxillary permanent lateral incisors are abnormally small and the coronal form is conical or peg-shaped.

d. Structure

147

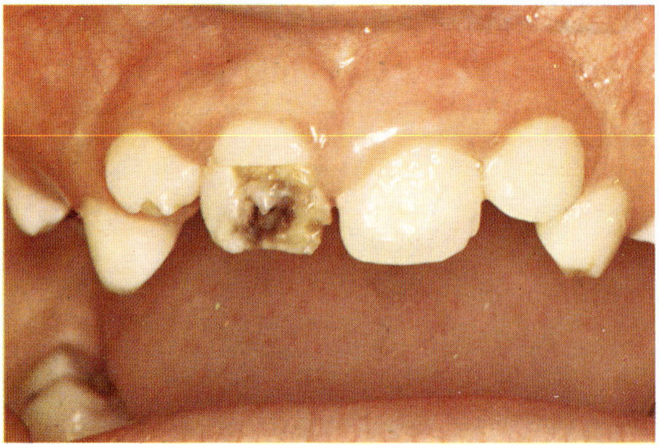

147 Localised enamel hypoplasia The marked enamel hypoplasia affecting the maxillary right permanent central incisor in this 9 year old boy was caused by severe trauma to the primary predecessor during the second year of life. Localised enamel defects of this type are described under the term 'Turner teeth' and show varying degrees of hypomineralisation or hypoplasia of the enamel.

148

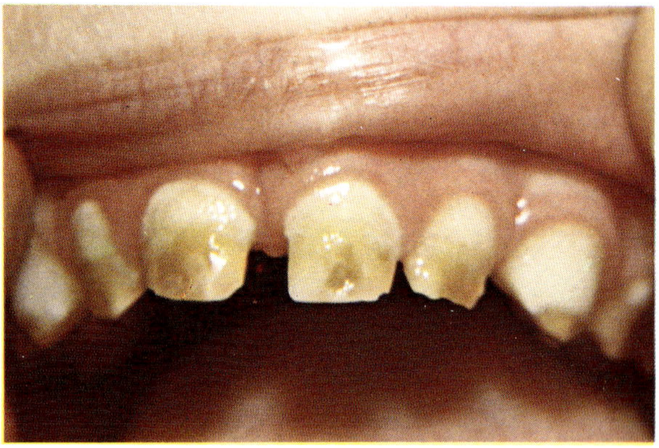

148 Prenatal enamel hypoplasia The marked enamel hypoplasia affecting the incisal two-thirds of the enamel on these maxillary primary incisors is evidence of a severe metabolic disturbance in foetal life, probably during the second and third trimesters of pregnancy. No cause for the condition was established in this patient. Similar defects are commonly seen in children with cerebral palsy.

149

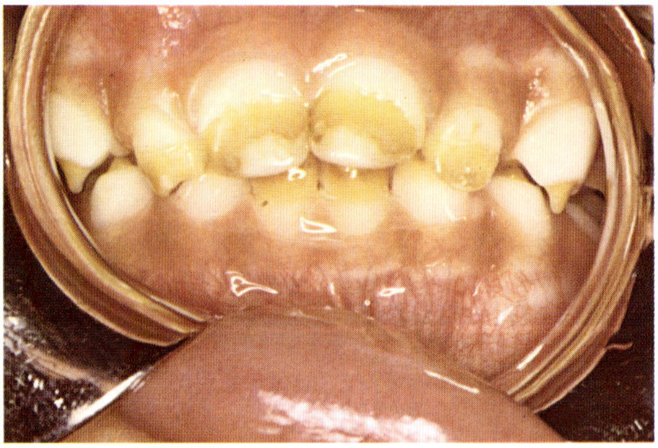

149 Neonatal enamel hypoplasia The wide band of enamel hypoplasia affecting the primary teeth in this child was associated with preterm birth and a birth weight of approximately 1.3kg. Low-birth-weight immature babies suffer considerable metabolic disturbance during the neonatal period and this is often reflected in defective amelogenesis.

150

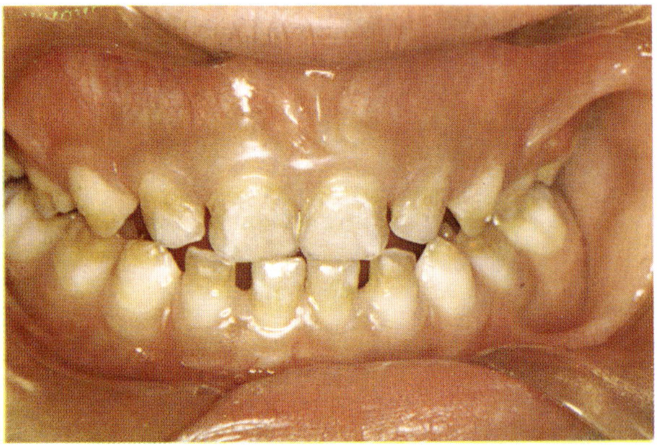

150 Neonatal enamel hypoplasia Premature birth combined with the neonatal exhibition of tetracycline antibiotics produced in this child a marked enamel hypoplasia combined with a yellowish-brown discolouration of the enamel and dentine in the primary dentition.

151

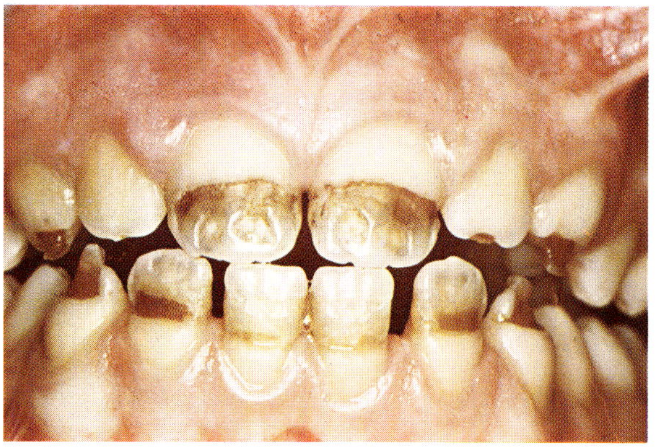

151 Infantile enamel hypoplasia A history of nutritional (vitamin D dependent) rickets during infancy probably accounts for the wide band of enamel hypoplasia affecting the maxillary permanent central incisors and canines and all the mandibular incisors and canines in this teenage girl. The later mineralisation of the maxillary lateral incisors explains the minimal defects on these teeth.

152

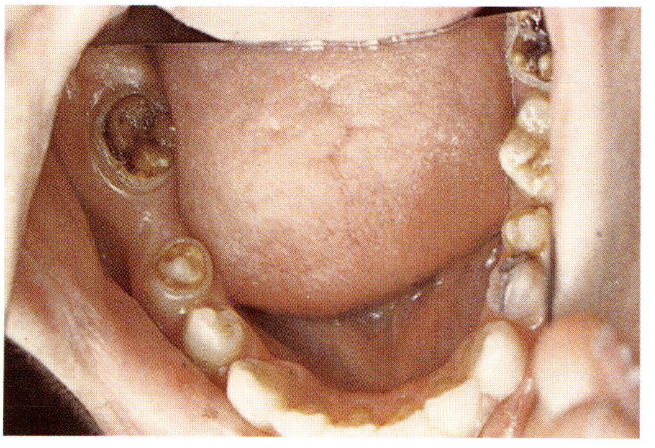

152 Enamel hypoplasia A severe attack of measles complicated by broncho-pneumonia during the fifth year of life may have been the cause of the chronological enamel hypoplasia affecting the mandibular second premolar and second molar in this teenage boy. Note that the earlier forming teeth are unaffected.

153

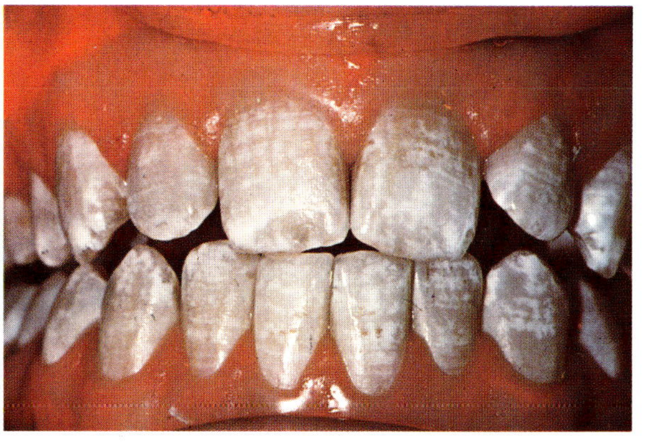

153 Fluorosis The consumption of both artificially fluoridated water and fluoride supplements during the formative period of the permanent teeth resulted in the generalised whitish mottling of the enamel seen in this teenager.

154

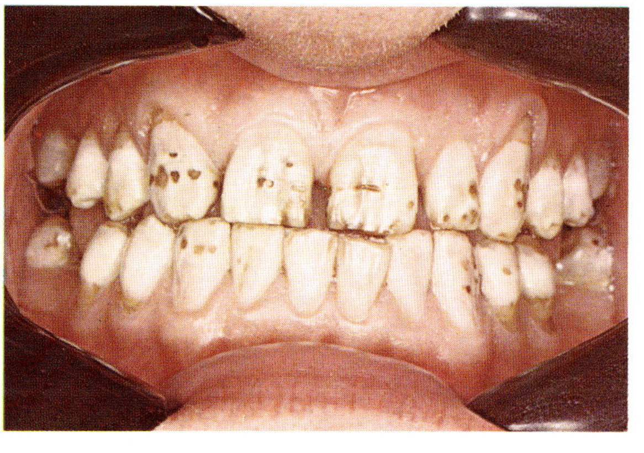

154 Endemic fluorosis This adolescent, who has been resident in a locality with a naturally high level of fluoride in the drinking water since birth, demonstrates localised areas of brown stained hypoplasia as well as generalised opaque brownish-white mottling of the enamel.

155 Amelogenesis imperfecta – thin and smooth hypoplasia type A markedly thin and smooth hypoplasia of the enamel is evident in this genetically determined autosomal dominant defect. Spacing of the teeth and either absence of, or few, carious lesions are two other features of this anomaly.

155

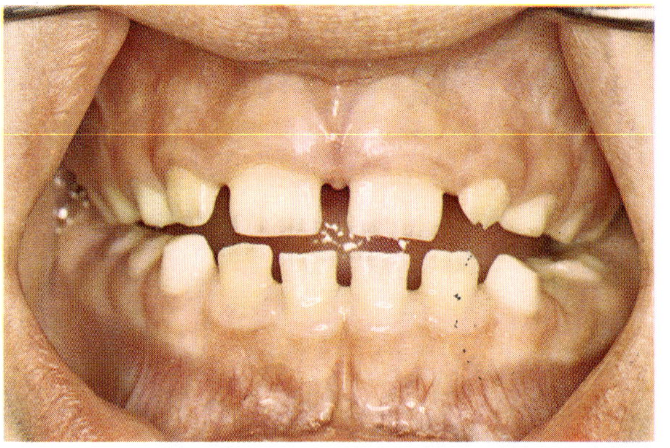

156, 157 Amelogenesis imperfecta – thin and smooth hypoplasia type Radiographs from another child with autosomal dominant thin and smooth enamel hypoplasia. Three of the radiographic features typical of this anomaly may be seen: difficulty in discerning the enamel, intrapulpal calcifications and coronal resorption of unerupted teeth.

156

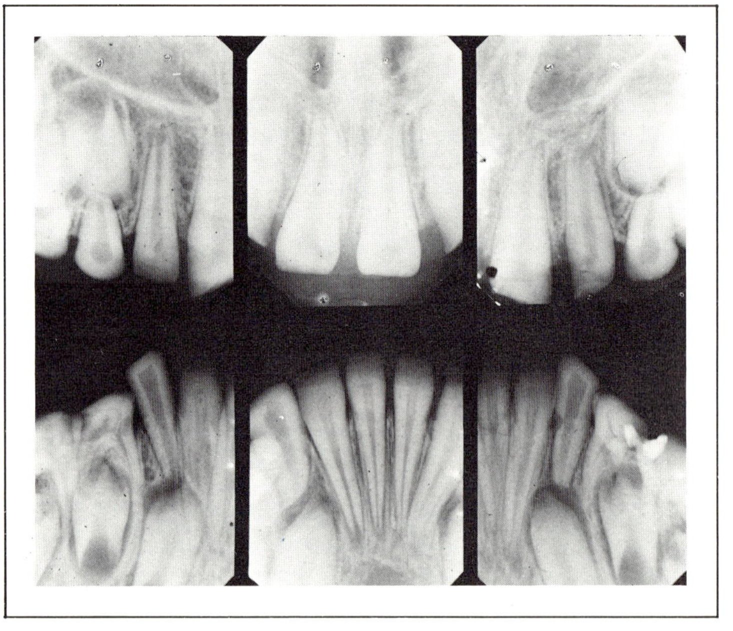

157

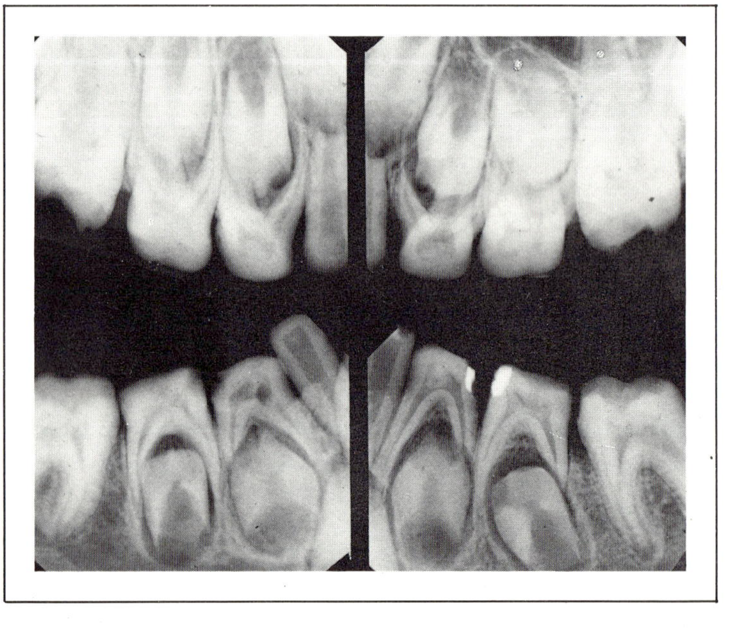

158

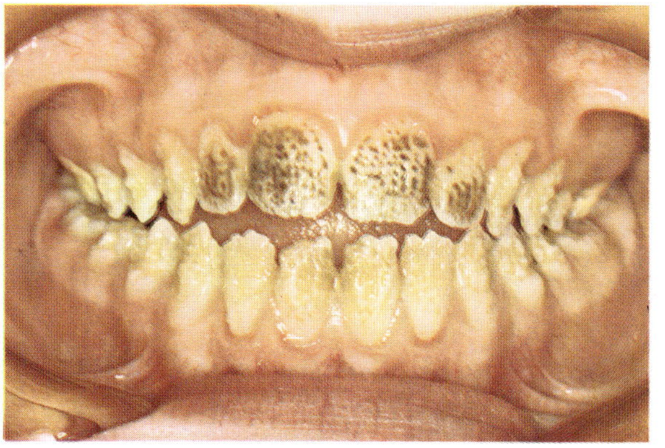

158 Amelogenesis imperfecta – randomly pitted hypoplasia type A generalised random pitting hypoplasia of the enamel is the characteristic feature of this autosomal dominant defect. The extrinsic brown stain deposited in the pits contributes to the cosmetic problem.

159

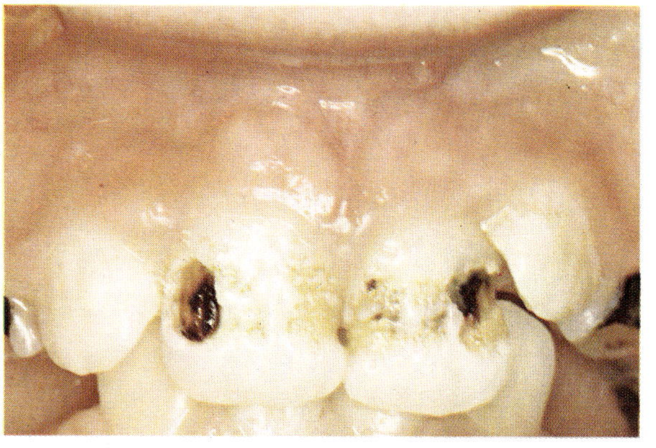

159 Amelogenesis imperfecta – localised hypoplasia type The wide band of localised enamel hypoplasia affecting the middle third of the labial enamel of these maxillary permanent central incisors was thought at first to have been caused by early trauma. The presence of a similar defect in other members of the family established the correct diagnosis for this autosomal dominant defect.

160

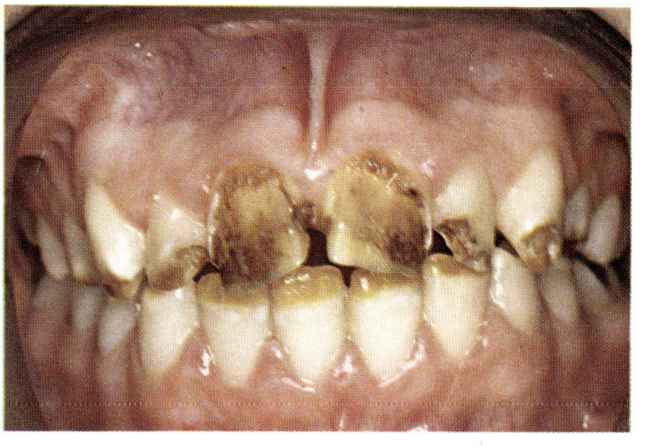

160 Amelogenesis imperfecta – hypocalcification type A curious variation in the degree of mineralisation of teeth, forming at the same age, is seen in this teenager with an autosomal dominantly determined hypocalcification of the enamel. Another feature of this anomaly is that the enamel in the cervical regions is more highly mineralised. Brownish staining of hypomineralised enamel is evident near to the incisal edges of the lower incisors, and considerable loss of soft enamel from the upper incisors has exposed the underlying sensitive dentine which is also stained a dark brown colour.

161

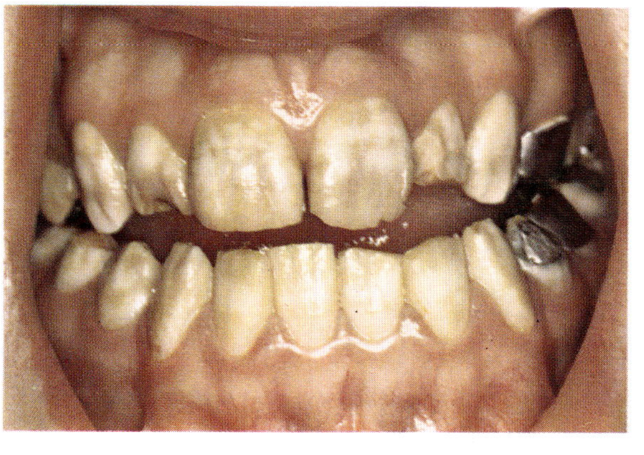

161 Amelogenesis imperfecta – hypomaturation type The brownish-white mottling of the enamel in this 12 year old girl is due to an X-linked recessively determined mineralising defect known as hypomaturation of the enamel. There is a tendency in the affected female for the enamel to be vertically banded by alternate columns of defective brownish enamel and normal white enamel. The relative softness of the tissue may be judged by the marked attrition of the upper lateral incisors.

162 Amelogenesis imperfecta – pigmented hypomaturation type The honey-coloured shiny enamel affecting all the permanent teeth in this 10 year old girl is typical of one of two types of autosomal recessive pigmented hypomaturation. A genetically determined enamel defect in which mineralisation of the enamel is defective.

162

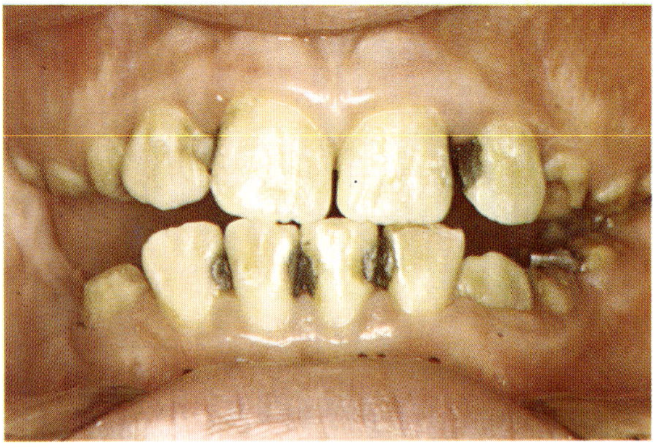

163 Amelogenesis imperfecta – pigmented hypomaturation type The chalky white teeth are characteristic of the second type of autosomal dominant pigmented hypomaturation of the enamel.

163

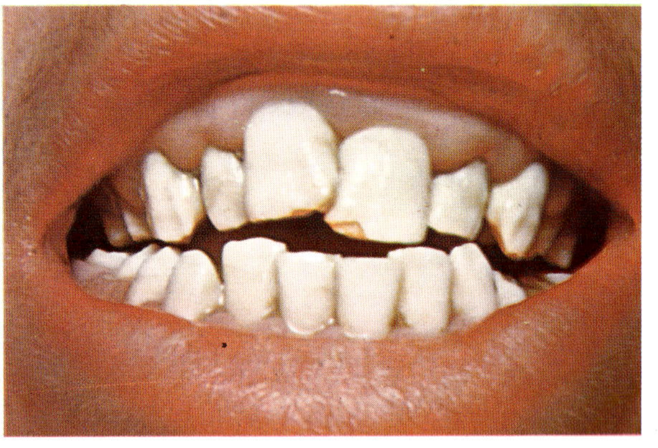

164 Amelogenesis imperfecta – snow-capped teeth A young boy exhibiting hypomineralised white patches on the incisal half of the enamel of the maxillary incisors. This type of genetically determined enamel hypomaturation has been given the term 'snow-capped' teeth.

164

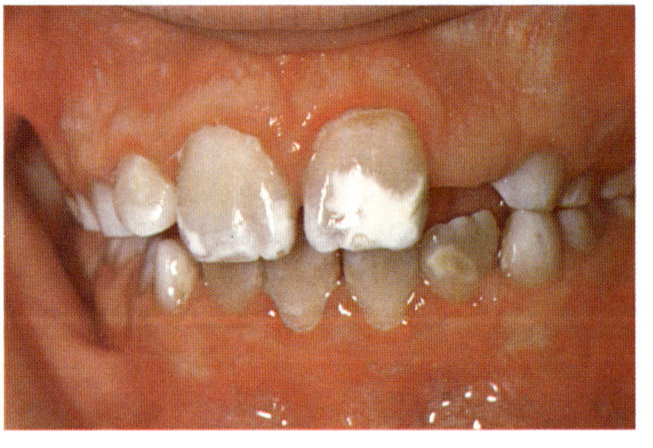

165 Amelogenesis imperfecta – hypomaturation-hypoplasia type associated with taurodontism The generalised opaquely mottled enamel of these permanent teeth is associated with occasional hypoplastic pitting in the cervical region of the crown and taurodontism. This adolescent girl is affected by a rare autosomal dominant defect of the enamel.

165

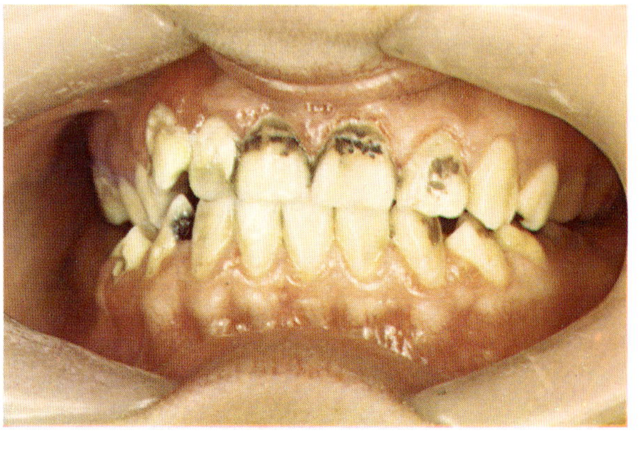

166

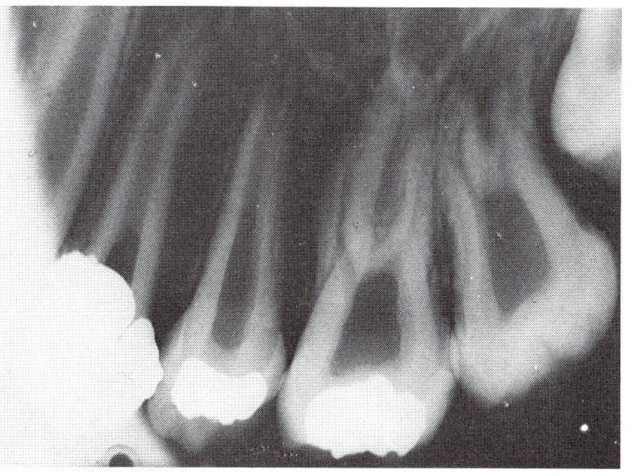

166 A radiograph of the case seen in **165** shows the characteristic lack of radiographic contrast between enamel and dentine, taurodontism of molars and generalised enlargement of the pulp spaces.

167

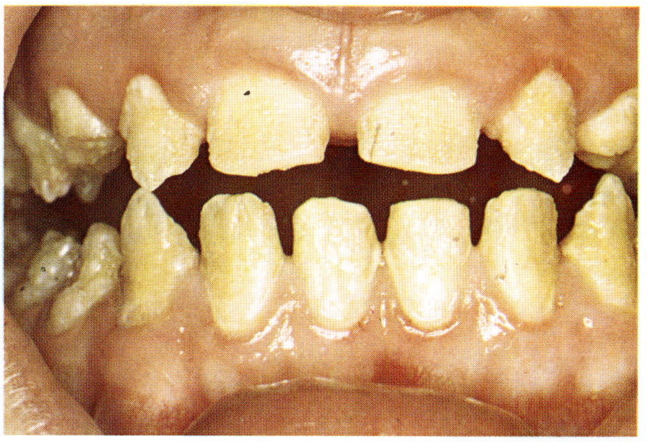

167 Epidermolysis bullosa dystrophica The generalised pitting hypoplasia of the enamel is associated in this boy with epidermolysis bullosa dystrophica. (See **463**)

168

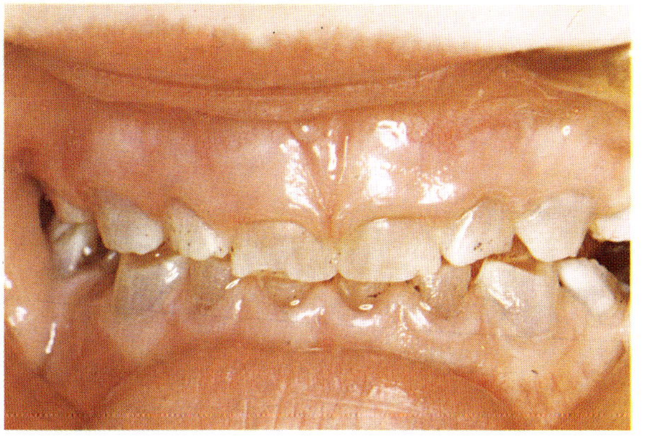

168 Dentinogenesis imperfecta (Hereditary opalescent dentine) The generalised brownish discolouration of the primary teeth in this young child is associated with an increased opalescence to transmitted light and a diminution in the size of the pulp spaces seen radiographically.

169

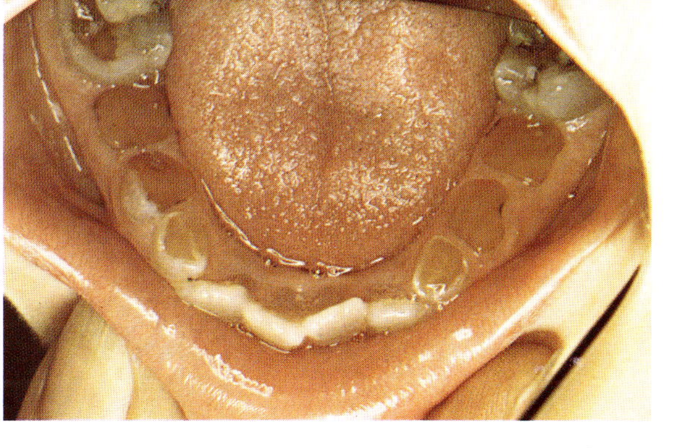

169 Dentinogenesis imperfecta (Hereditary opalescent dentine) The gross attrition of these mandibular primary canines and molars shows the typical amber-brown colour of the exposed dentine. Note that despite the extreme wear on these teeth there is no clinical exposure of the pulp space.

170 Dentinogenesis imperfecta (Hereditary opalescent dentine) The permanent teeth in this teenager show the characteristic bluish-brown discolouration and the bulbous deformity of the crowns. Attrition is already evident on all the incisor teeth.

170

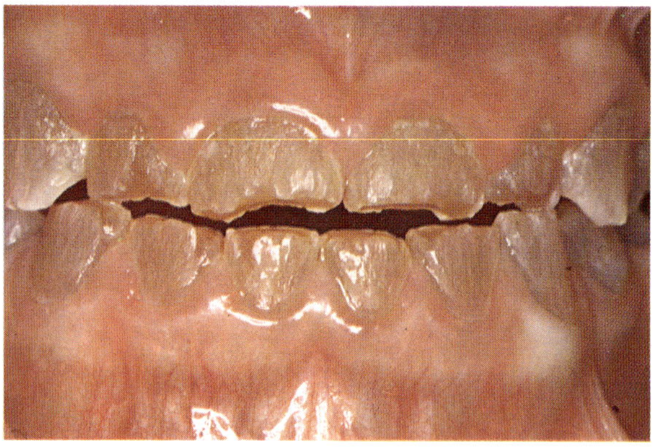

171 Dentinogenesis imperfecta (Hereditary opalescent dentine) The thin greyish enamel covering this 8 year old boy's incisors is associated with a severe genetically determined dentine defect. Mandibular incisal attrition is already advanced.

171

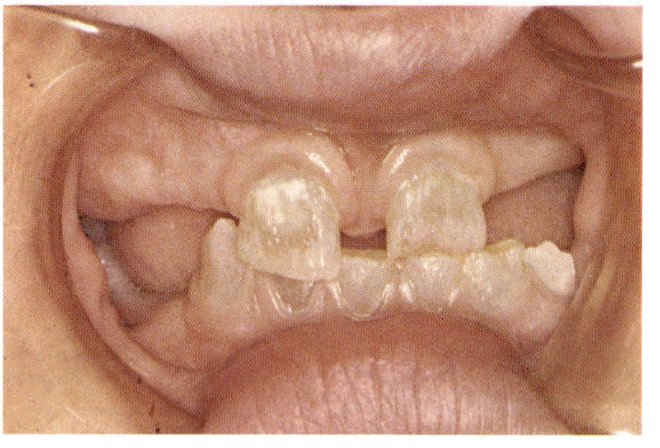

172 Radiographs of the case seen in **171** show the typical calcific obliteration of the pulp chambers of recently erupted teeth.

172

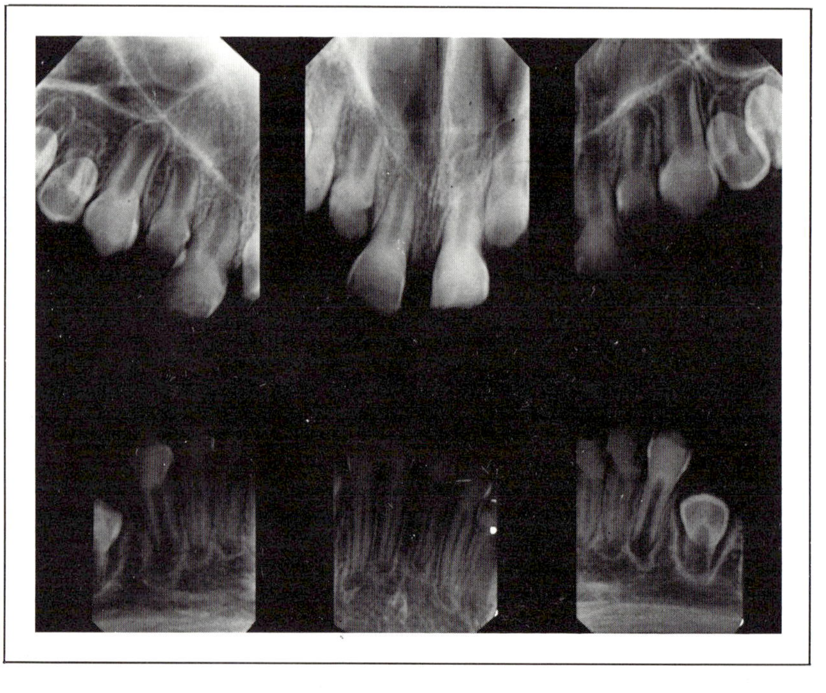

173 Dentinogenesis imperfecta (Hereditary opalescent dentine) The rapid attrition so often a feature of this hereditary defect may be seen affecting the mandibular first permanent molars. The recently erupted premolars do not yet show this abnormal wear pattern.

173

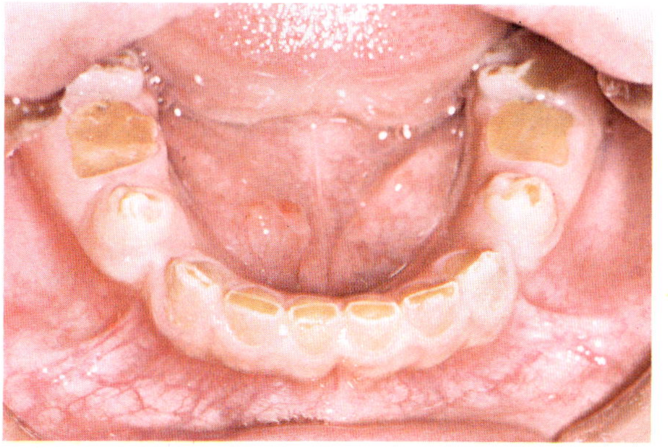

174 Coronal dentine dysplasia The colour and shape of teeth in this autosomal dominant defect of dentine formation are within normal limits. Apart from some early incisal attrition the teeth might be considered clinically normal.

174

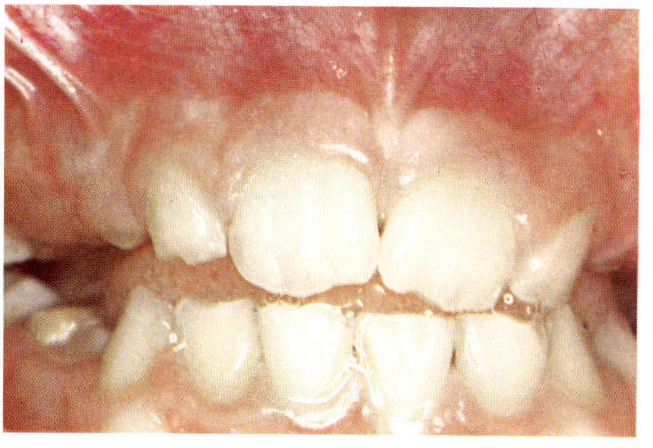

175 Further abnormalities of the case seen in **174** are evident in the radiograph. This shows the characteristic flame-shaped coronal pulp chambers and almost complete obliteration of the root canals. In some teeth a portion of the flame-shaped pulp chamber is occupied by a calcific pulp stone.

175

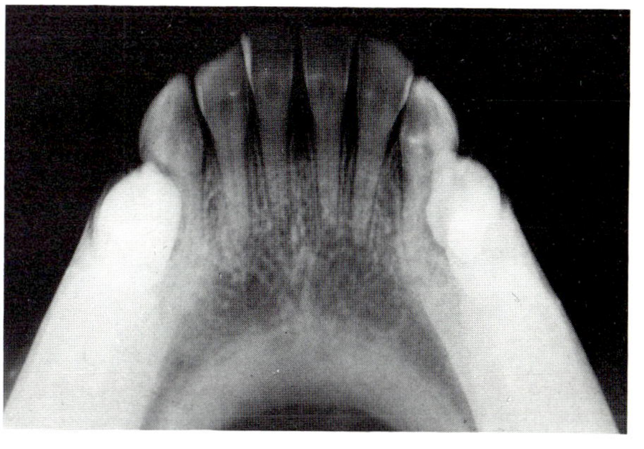

176 Osteogenesis imperfecta The bluish-brown discolouration of the mandibular primary central incisors in this infant with osteogenesis imperfecta is evidence of the occasional association of this generalised bony defect with dentinogenesis imperfecta. (See **54** and **477**)

176

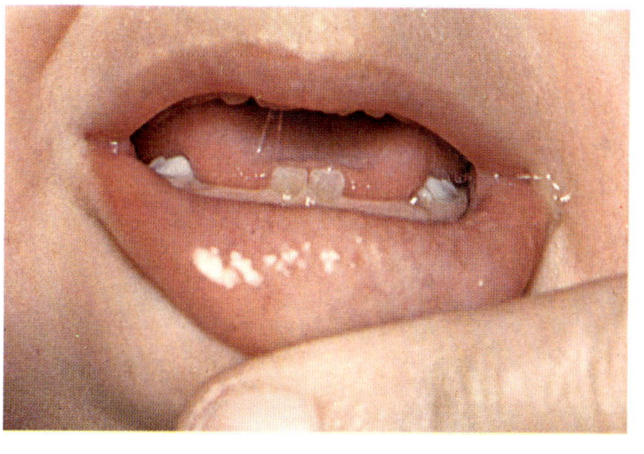

177

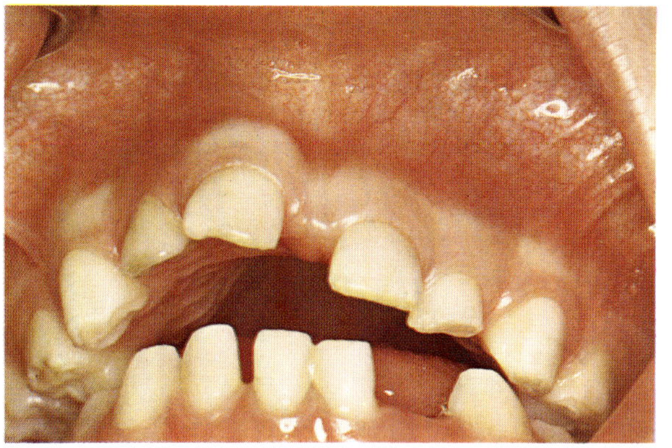

177 Vitamin D resistant rickets The mandibular left primary lateral incisor in this 4 year old boy with vitamin D resistant rickets was extracted after it became abscessed.

178

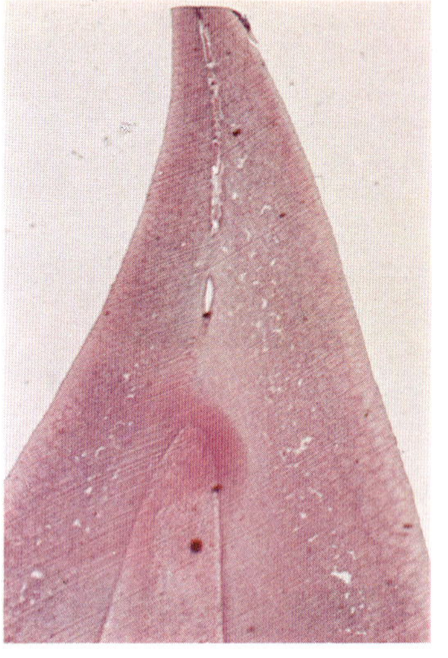

178 Examination of an histological section of the tooth described in **177** shows developmental defects in the dentine leading to the pulpal horns. It is probable that following attrition of the incisal enamel, infection gained access to the pulp via these dentinal defects. (See **141**, **142** and **478**) (×20)

179

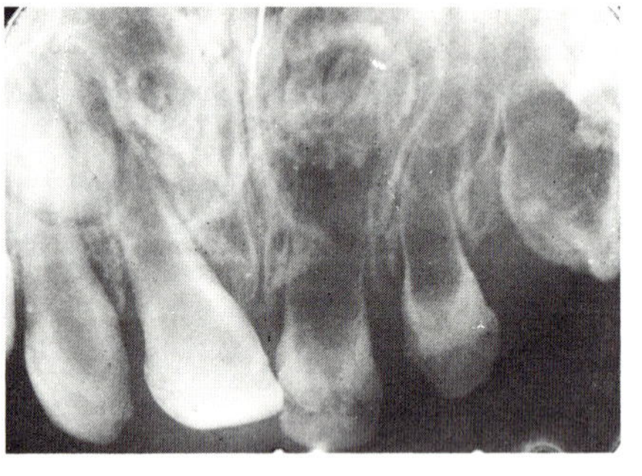

179 Odontodysplasia Radiograph of a child aged 2 years showing the 'ghost-like' appearance of the maxillary left primary incisors and canine affected by odontodysplasia.

180

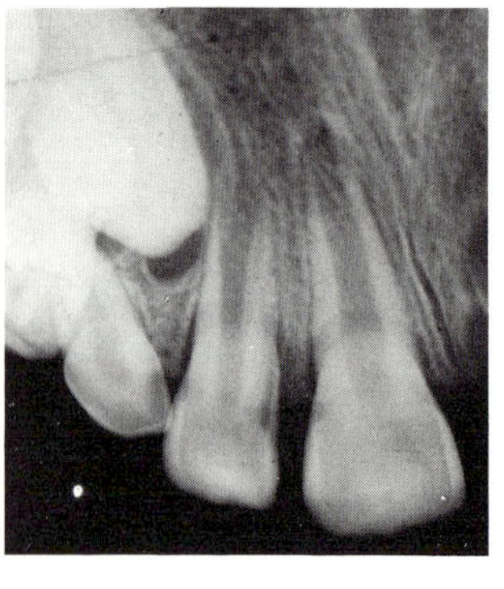

181

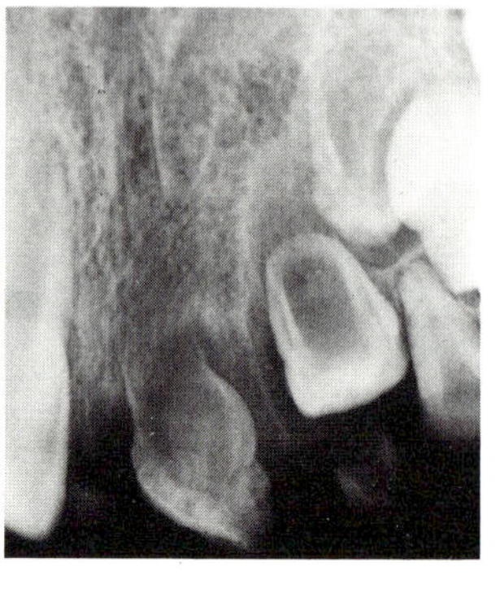

180, 181 Odontodysplasia The gross developmental anomaly of teeth affected by odontodysplasia is seen in these radiographs. While the permanent teeth on the right side of the maxilla appear to be developing normally, those on the left have a 'ghost-like' appearance. The left lateral incisor is delayed in its eruption.

e. Colour

182

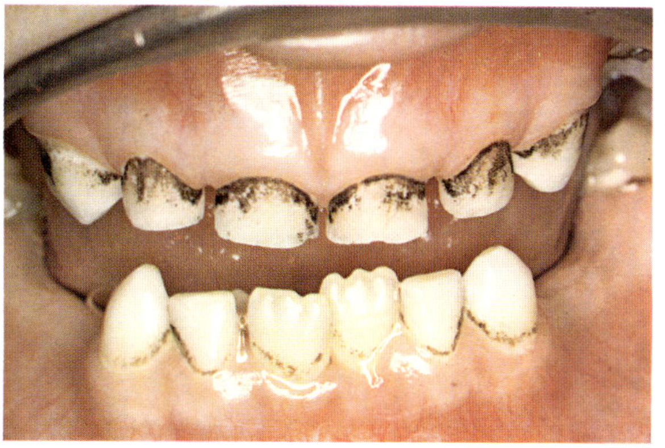

182 Black stain The black extrinsic stain in this young child is limited to the cervical areas of the labial surfaces of the maxillary primary incisors and canines. The recent consumption of iron medicine for a nutritional anaemia was probably the aetiological agent.

183

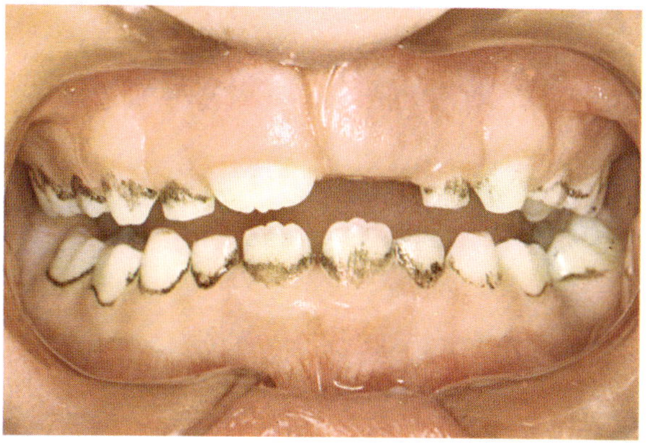

183 Black stain The dark brownish-black extrinsic stain in this 7 year old is seen characteristically covering the cervical regions of the crowns on most of the teeth. The term 'mesenteric line' has been given to this condition which is frequently associated with a low caries incidence.

184

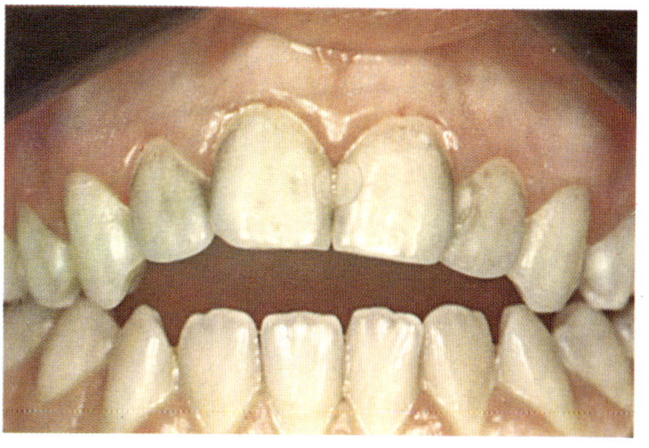

184 Green stain Dental plaque covering the labial surfaces of the upper anterior teeth in this teenage girl is discoloured green by the growth of chromogenic bacteria. Such deposits tend to recur after removal; this may be due to roughening of the enamel surface by early demineralisation.

185

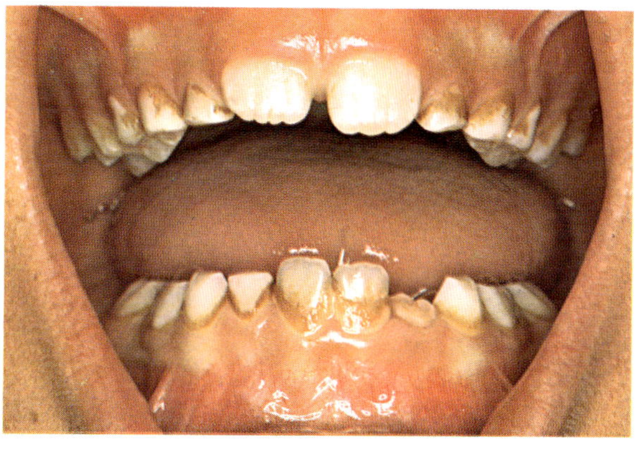

185 Orange stain The cervical plaque in this 7 year old is orange in colour and affects all the teeth except for the recently erupted maxillary permanent central incisors. This type of extrinsic stain is often associated with poor oral hygiene.

186

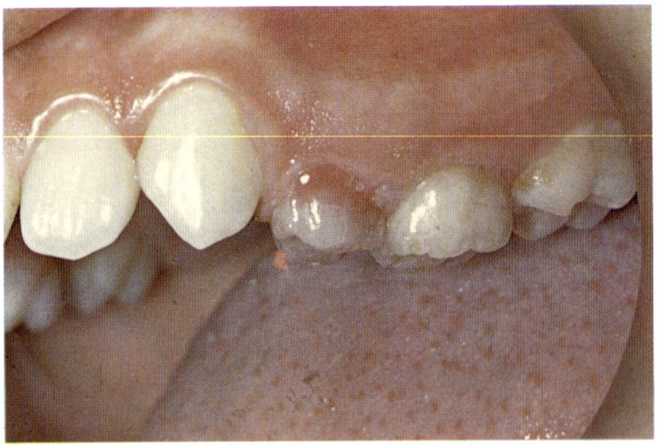

186 Physiological resorption The pinkish discolouration of the maxillary first primary molar is associated with advanced physiological resorption involving the coronal tissues. The tooth was exfoliated shortly afterwards.

187

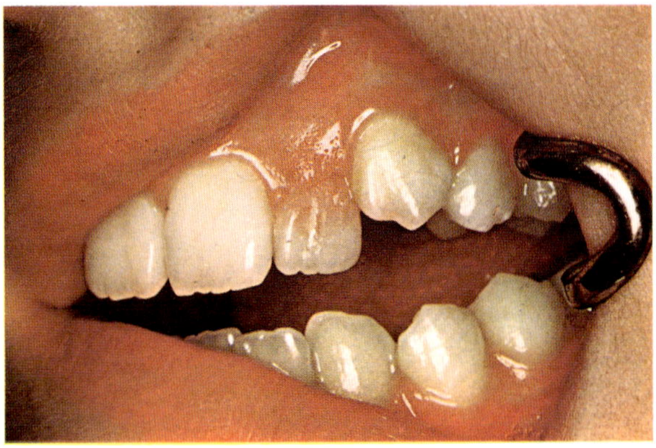

187 Pink spot The intrinsic pinkish-red discolouration of the maxillary left permanent lateral incisor is due to marked internal coronal resorption. The cause of the pathological resorption is unknown.

188

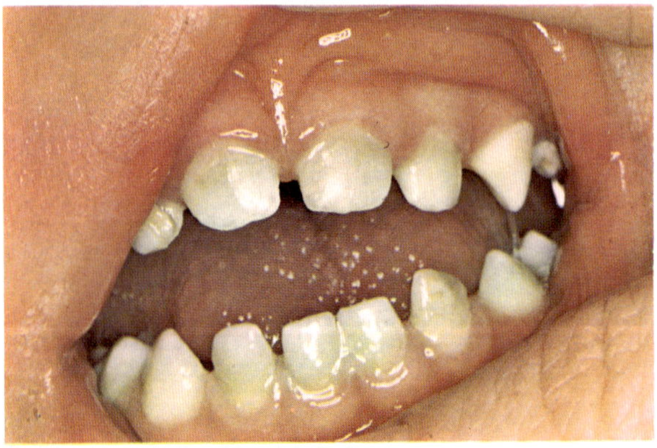

188 Icterus gravis neonatorum The intrinsic greenish discolouration of the primary dentition in this young child was associated with severe jaundice (hyperbilirubinaemia) in the first few days of life.

189

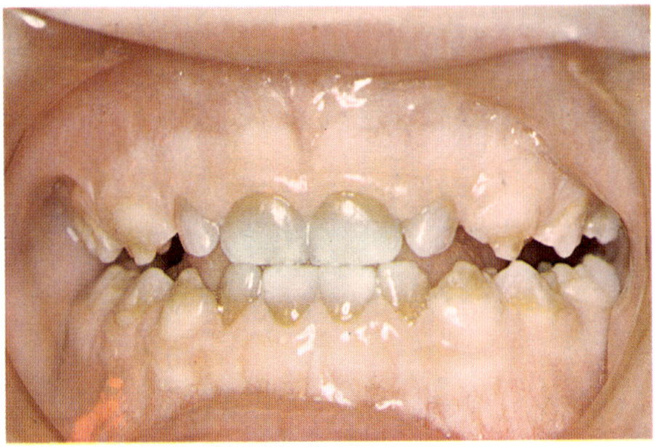

189 Tetracycline stain When only 10 days old this child developed a severe staphylococcal skin and conjunctival infection for which tetracycline therapy was given for a week. The dental hard tissues formed during this period are stained a golden-brown colour. Note also the neonatal enamel hypoplasia which is principally affecting the primary canines.

190, 191, 192 Tetracycline stain The intrinsic staining of teeth affecting the permanent dentition of all these children is associated with a considerable ingestion of tetracycline drugs during early childhood. The colour varies from yellow-brown, to bluish-grey and finally to greyish-brown.

190

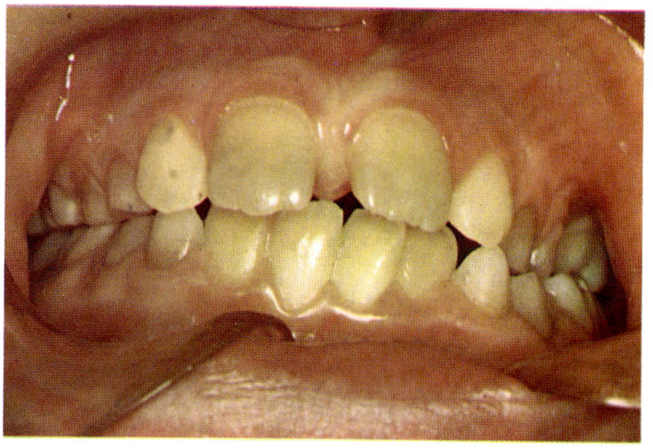

191

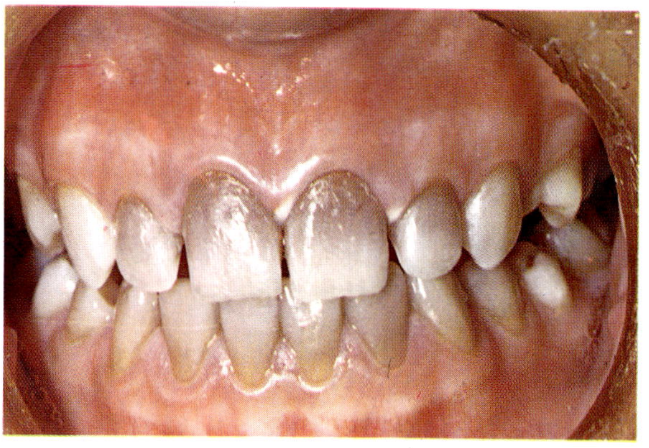

192

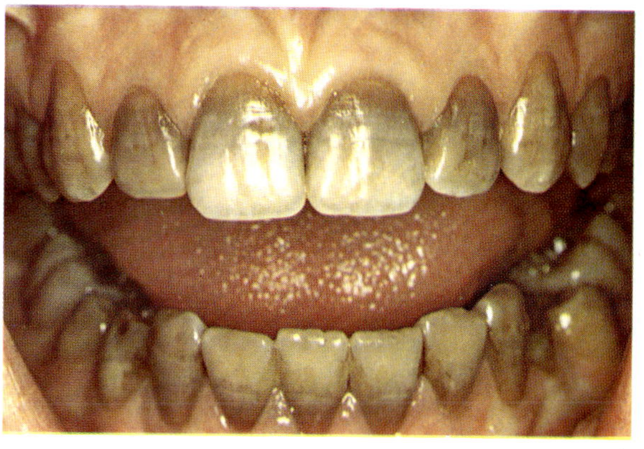

193 Tetracycline stain Prolonged tetracycline therapy for cystic fibrosis has produced the most severe form of discolouration. In this case a distinct generalised chronological enamel hypoplasia is evident. Whether this was caused by a toxic effect of the antibiotic or the metabolic disturbance of the illness is uncertain.

193

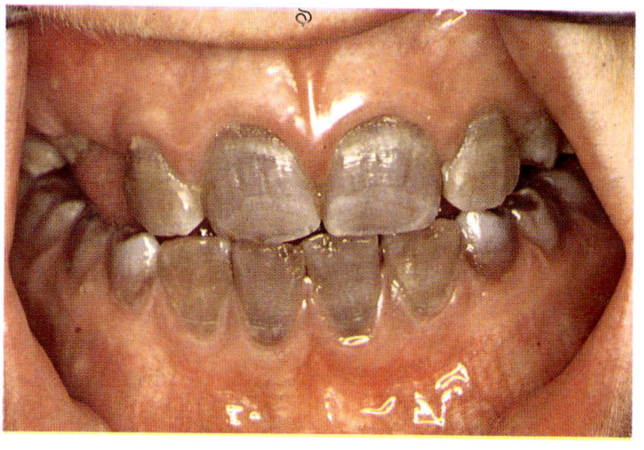

194

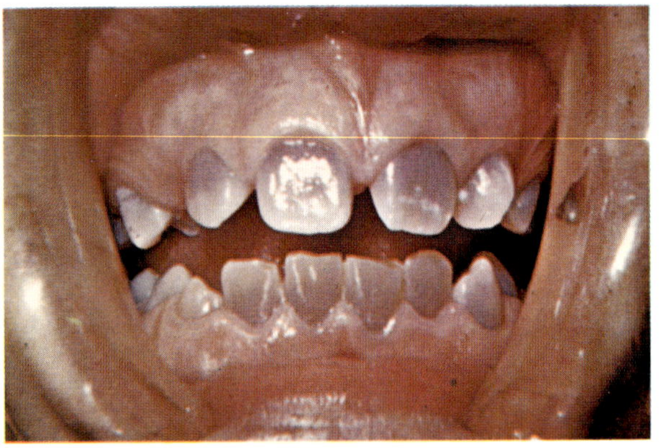

194 Dentinogenesis imperfecta (Hereditary opalescent dentine) Characteristic bluish-grey discolouration of the permanent teeth in a child with hereditary opalescent dentine.

195

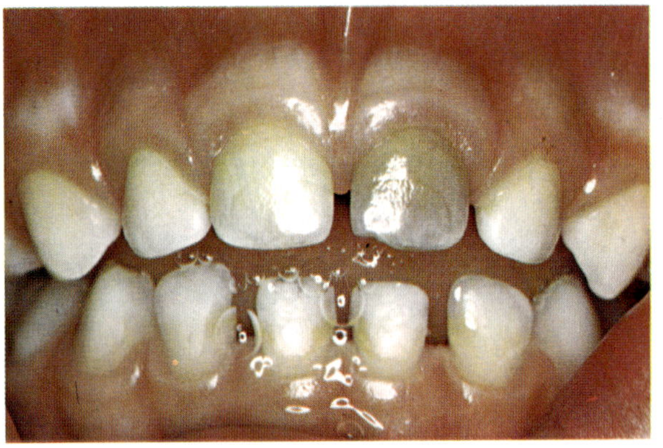

195 Pulpal necrosis – primary dentition The greyish discolouration of the maxillary left central incisor is associated with a non-vital pulp. The slight loss of enamel on the incisal edge suggests the possibility of previous trauma.

196

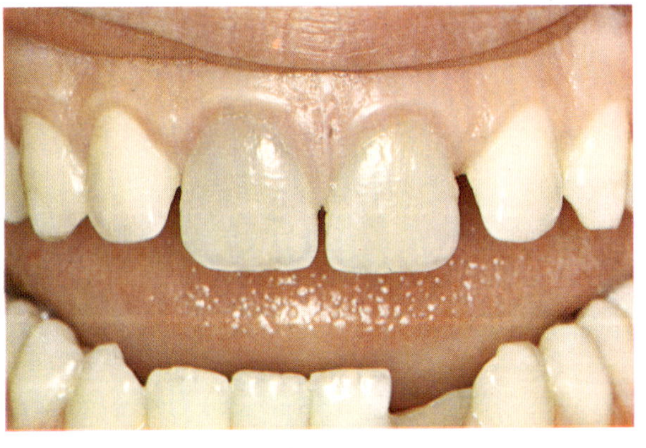

196 Pulpal necrosis – permanent dentition The greyish discolouration of the maxillary central incisors in this child was noted two years after an accident in which the lower left lateral incisor was avulsed. The teeth did not respond to vitality tests and the pulps were found to be necrotic.

f. Eruption/exfoliation

197

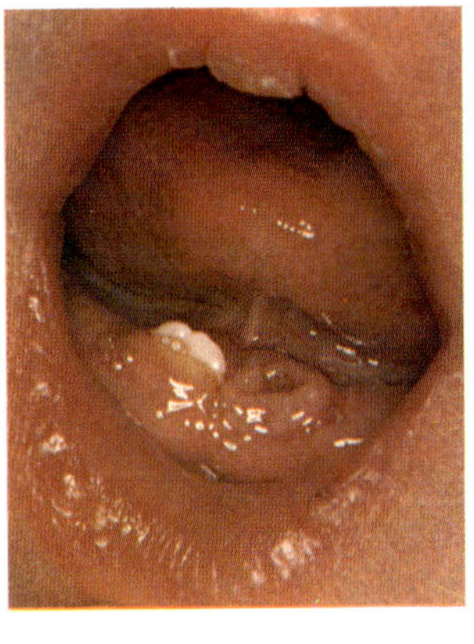

197 Natal teeth This neonate was noted to have two mandibular primary incisors erupted at birth. One was removed just prior to the photograph being taken; the other was extremely mobile and was also removed to avoid the possibility of accidental inhalation.

198

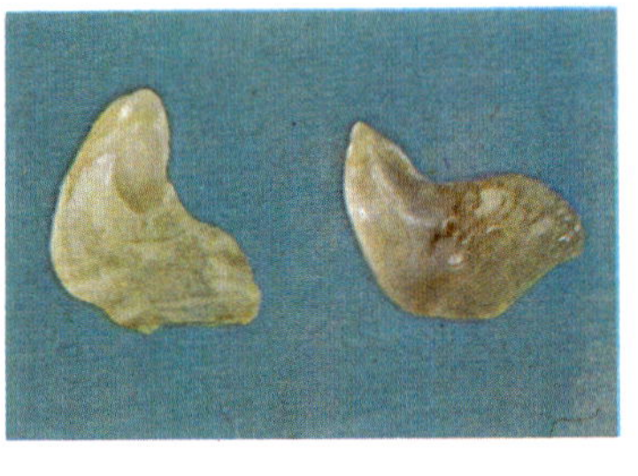

198 Examination of the teeth described in **197** showed poorly mineralised enamel and dilacerated crowns associated with very little root formation.

199 Neonatal teeth The mandibular primary central incisors in this baby erupted soon after birth. The radiograph confirms that the teeth are not supplementals. Extraction of such teeth at an early age may disrupt the occlusion in the lower arch.

199

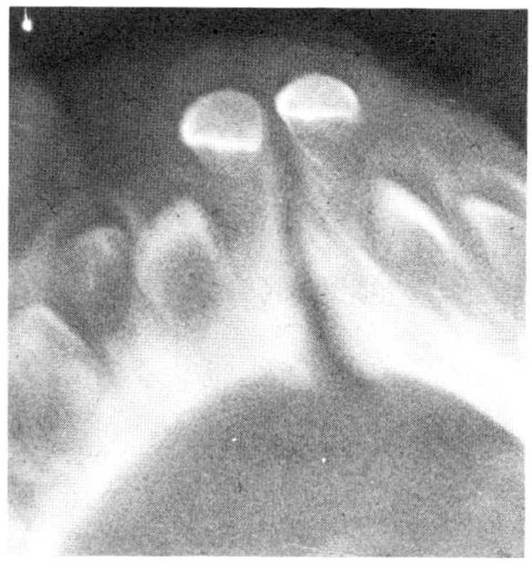

200 Ectopic eruption – first permanent molar This radiograph shows the ectopic eruption and impaction of the maxillary first permanent molar associated with advanced resorption of the second primary molar. Considerable crowding of teeth in the arch can be expected in such cases.

200

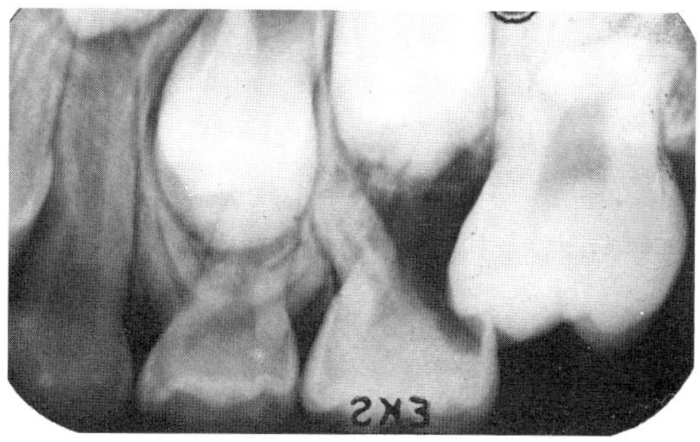

201 Ectopic eruption – permanent lateral incisor Ectopic eruption of the maxillary right permanent lateral incisor in this radiograph is associated with advanced root resorption of the adjacent primary canine.

201

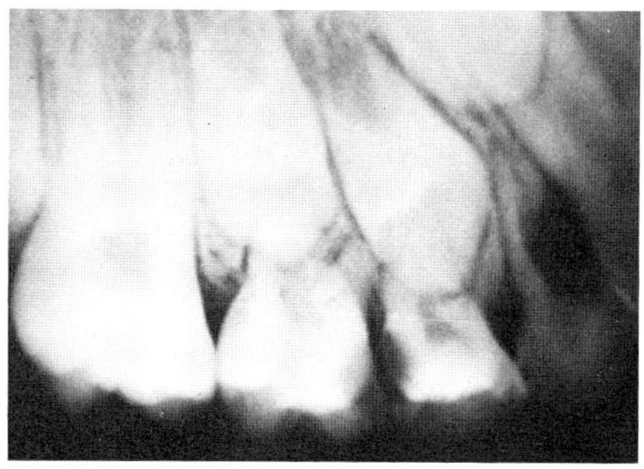

202 Ectopic eruption – permanent canine Ectopic eruption and impaction of the maxillary right permanent canine may be seen to be involved with advanced resorption of the lateral incisor root and early resorption of the central incisor root apex.

202

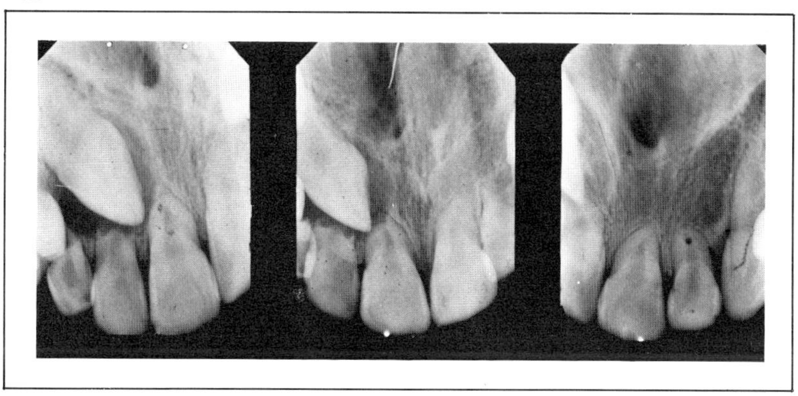

203 Ectopic eruption – permanent canine The swelling in the lower labial sulcus of this 10 year old child is due to an ectopically erupting permanent left canine.

203

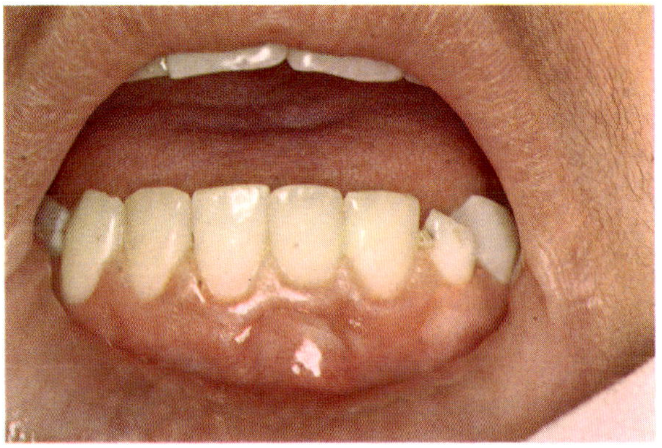

204 Delayed eruption – maxillary permanent central incisor Prolonged delay in the eruption of permanent teeth is commonly seen in the premaxillary region. It suggests the necessity for adequate radiographic examination to confirm the presence of the teeth and to rule out the possibility of supernumeraries, dilacerations, odontomes and cysts etc.

204

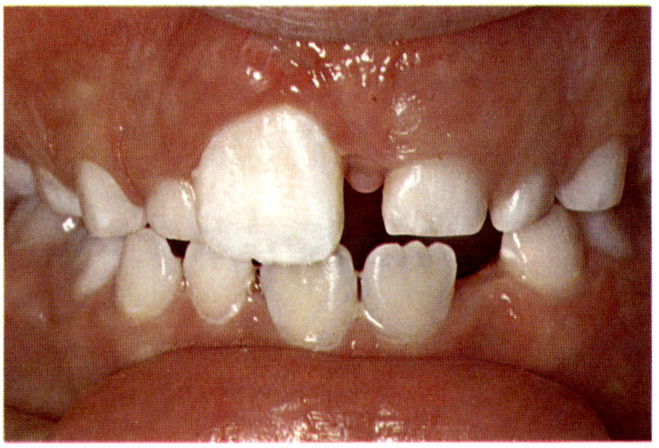

205 Delayed eruption – permanent central incisor, due to presence of mesiodens This radiograph shows that the retained maxillary left primary central incisor is associated with a mesiodens and delayed eruption of the overlying permanent central incisor. Extraction of the primary tooth and surgical removal of the mesiodens resulted in eruption of the permanent successor.

205

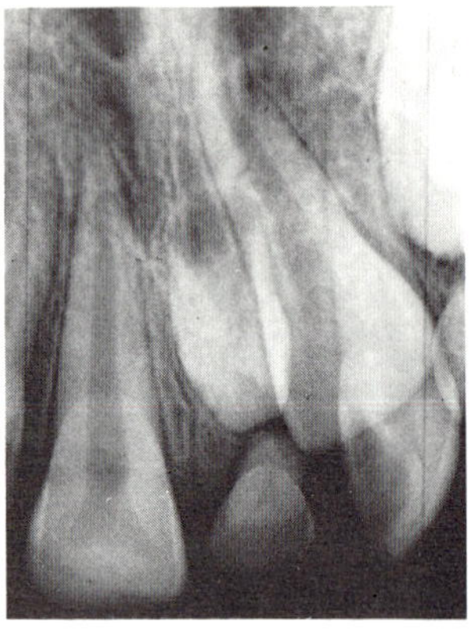

206 Delayed eruption – permanent incisor, due to chronic dentoalveolar infection This radiograph shows the retained cariously involved maxillary left primary central incisor associated with a large periapical area of rarefaction, incomplete root resorption and delayed eruption of the overlying permanent central incisor. Extraction of the primary tooth resulted in eruption of the permanent successor.

206

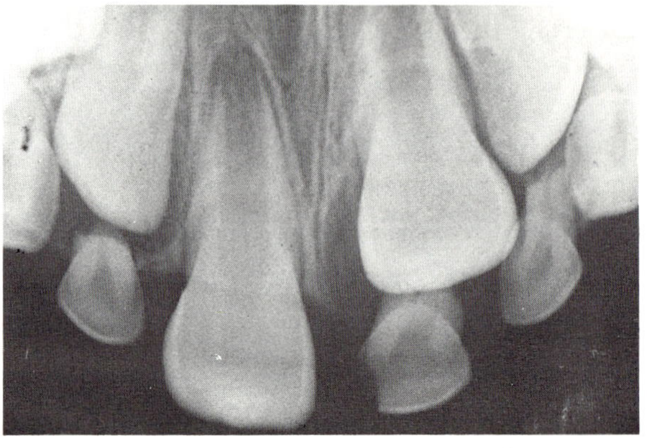

207 Retained primary teeth Eruption of mandibular permanent incisors lingual to the primary incisors is occasionally associated with abnormal root resorption of the primary incisors. In these circumstances extraction of the primary teeth is necessary to allow the permanent successors to attain their normal position within the arch.

207

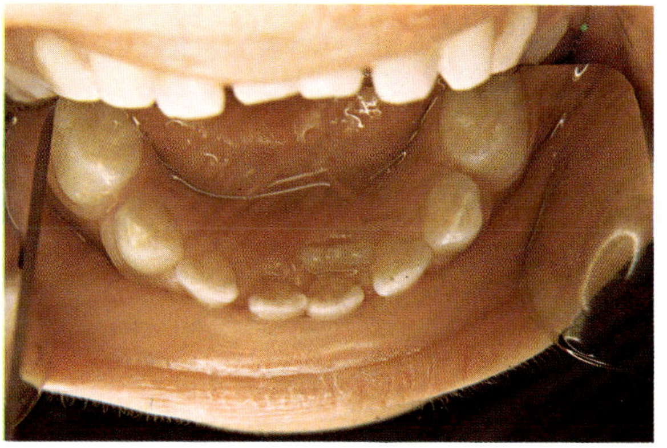

208 Rotated tooth germ The unerupted mandibular second premolar is both distally inclined and rotated. Maintenance of arch length by means of a space maintainer may allow this tooth to align and upright itself as it continues to erupt.

208

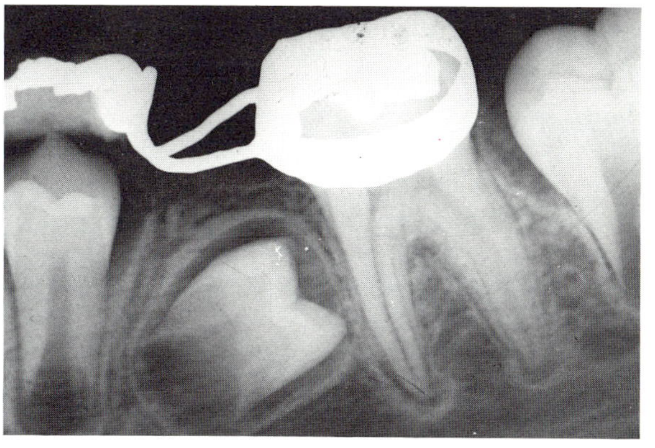

209 Bilateral infraocclusion (Submergence) – primary molars Infraocclusion (submergence) of primary molars, as seen affecting the mandibular second primary molars in this child, may or may not be associated with the congenital absence of the underlying premolars. Ankylosis of the primary tooth, a constant feature, may be diagnosed by percussion of the crown which evokes a characteristically dull sound.

209

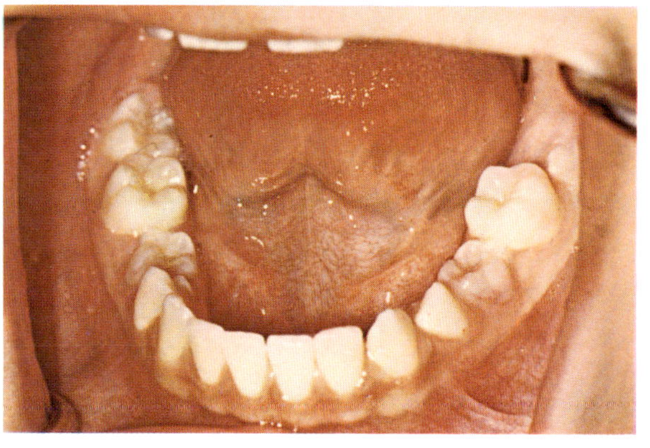

210 Unilateral infraocclusion (Submergence) – primary molars A radiograph of an infraoccluded mandibular second primary molar shows the presence of the underlying premolar and suggests the possibility of ankylosis. Mesial tipping of the first permanent molar is evident with associated loss of arch length and vertical impaction of the infraoccluded primary molar.

210

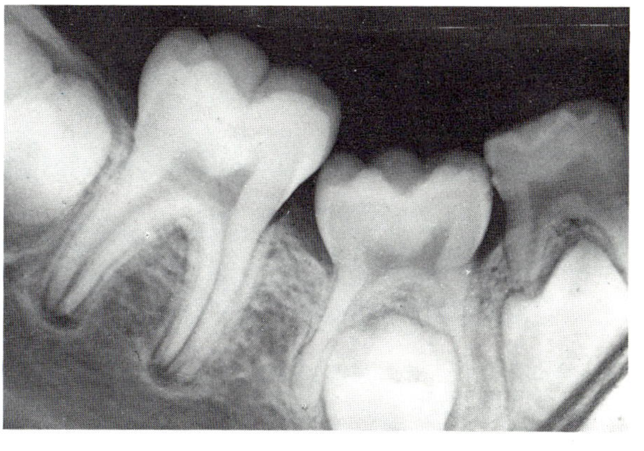

211

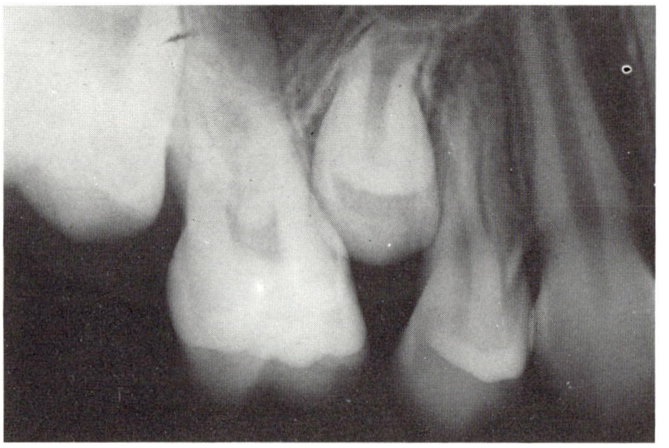

211 Early loss – primary molar The premature extraction of a grossly carious maxillary second primary molar in this child without subsequent space maintenance allowed the mesial movement of the first permanent molar. The radiograph demonstrates the loss of arch length and the vertical impaction of the second premolar.

212

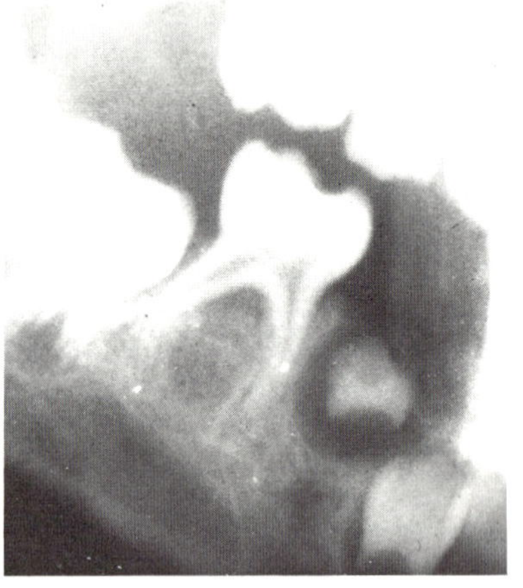

212 Developmental arrest of permanent tooth germ A bony hard swelling was present on the buccal aspect of the alveolus in the site of a previously extracted mandibular right first primary molar in this 4 year old boy. A radiograph of the right jaw shows evidence of developmental arrest of the first premolar tooth germ associated with a surrounding area of bony rarefaction. This is an uncommon sequel to longstanding, untreated pulpal infection in a primary tooth.

213

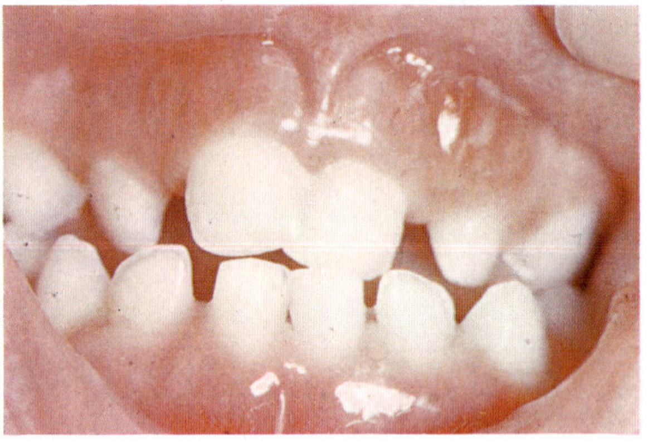

213 Papillon-Lefèvre syndrome (Hyperkeratosis palmoplantaris with periodontosis) The swollen, shiny-red gingivae in this $2\frac{1}{2}$ year old girl with mobile and overlapping maxillary central incisors are features of this syndrome.

214

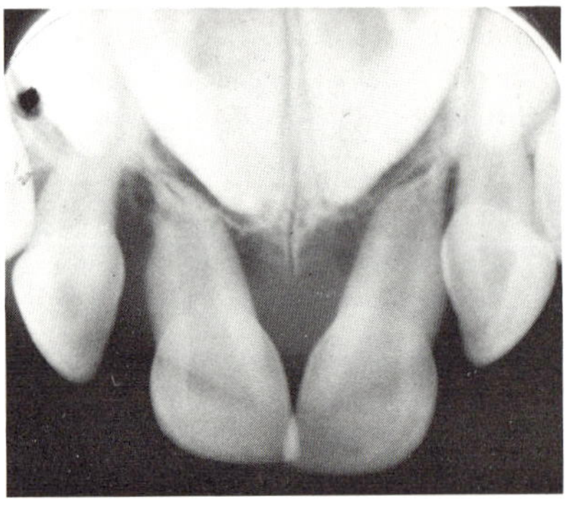

214 The radiograph of the upper incisor region of the child shown in **213** confirms the gross loss of alveolar bony support for the primary teeth which were shed shortly afterwards. The condition is transmitted as an autosomal recessive genetic defect. (See **462**)

215, 216 Hypophosphatasia At the age of 2 years 4 months a female homozygote with autosomal recessive hypophosphatasia has already lost all her mandibular primary incisors and the left maxillary canine is excessively loose. Radiographs show gross loss of bony alveolar support around all the erupted teeth and large pulp chambers in the primary molars.

215

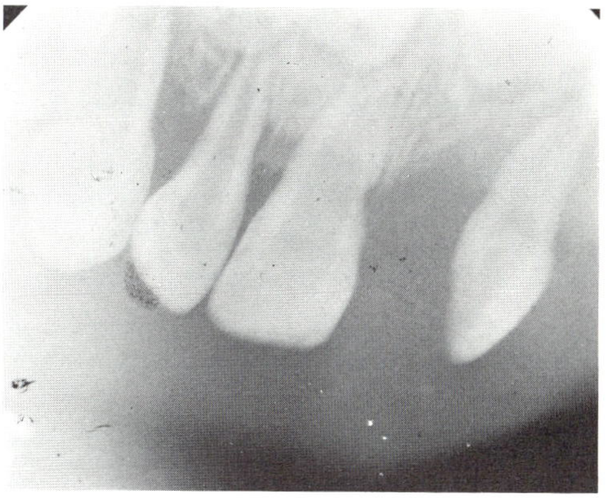

216

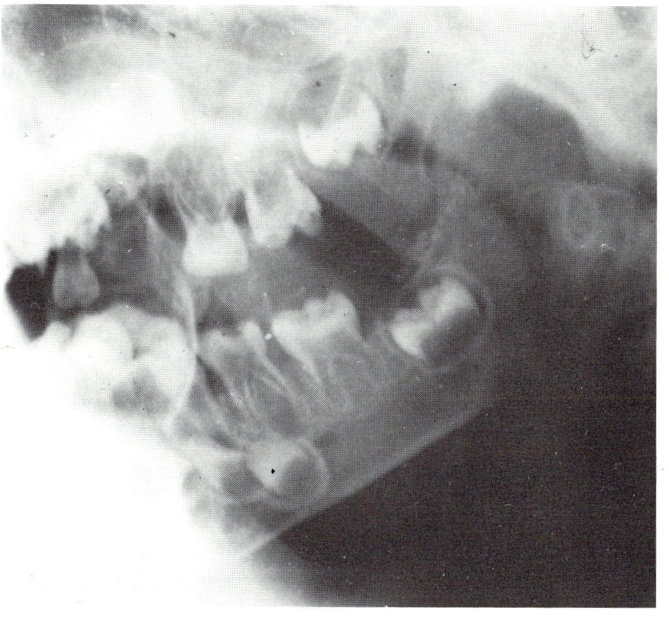

217 Histological section of the maxillary canine seen in **215** and **216** shows a pathognomonic absence of cementum on the surface of the root dentine which is covered by a layer of bacterial plaque. (×50)

217

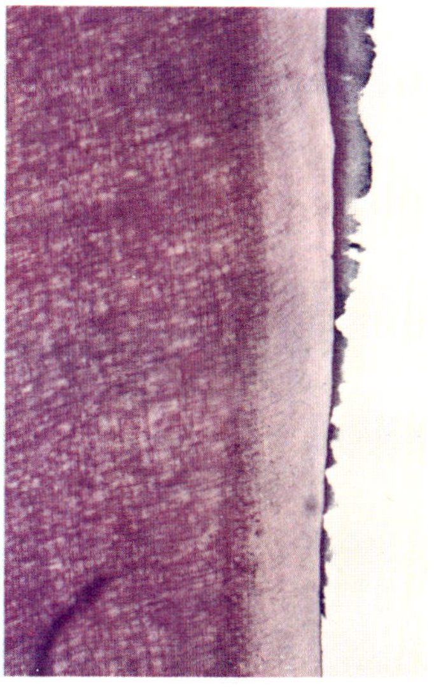

218, 219 Histiocytosis X (Hand-Schüller-Christian type) The sequestrating maxillary first permanent molars are at the centre of grossly destructive lesions of mucosa and bone in this 3 year old girl. The right first permanent molar and the palatal root of the second primary molar are exposed by necrotic ulceration of tissue, while on the left side the palatal aspects of these teeth are covered by tissue resembling bright red granulations.

218

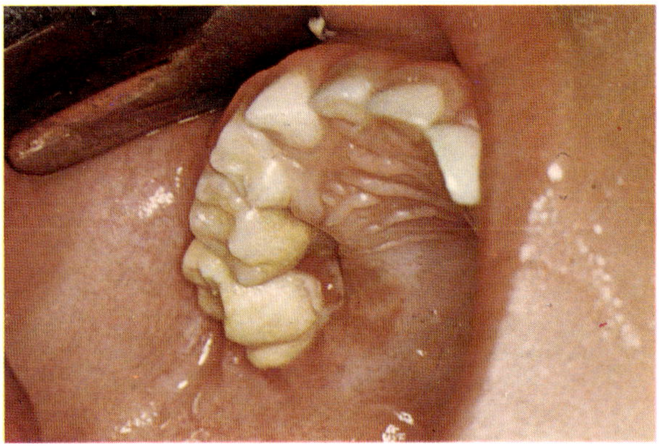

219

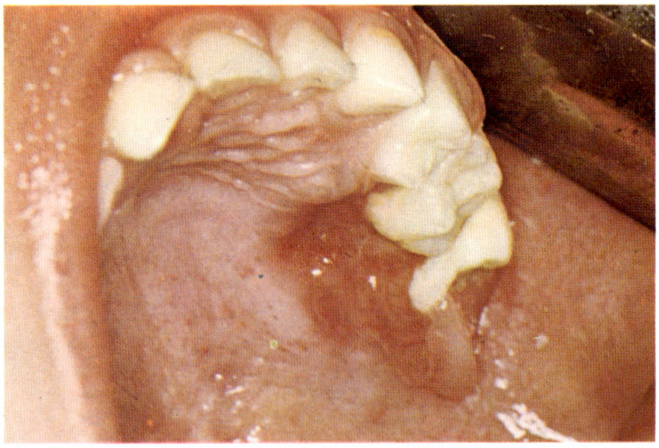

220 The radiograph of the child seen in **218** and **219** shows the typical 'punched-out' osteolytic lesion of bone involving the mandibular second primary molar.

220

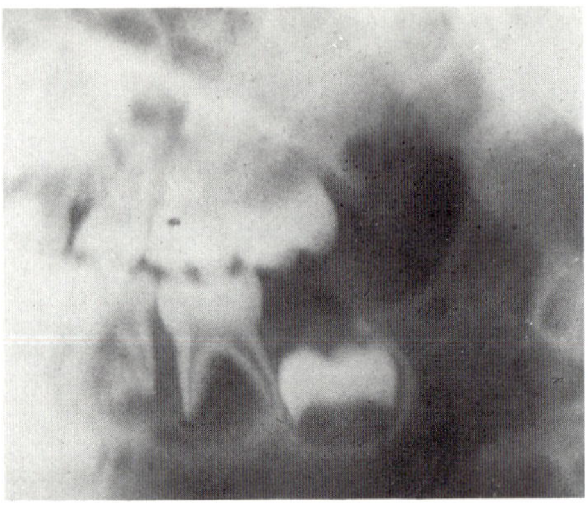

g. Trauma

(i) Primary dentition

221 Intrusion Bilateral intrusion of maxillary central incisors resulting from a fall 18 hours previously.

221

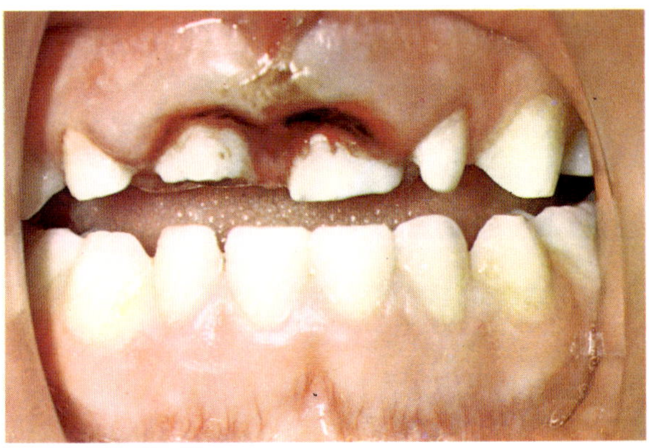

222 Pulpal necrosis The greyish coronal discolouration seen in the maxillary right central incisor is typical of teeth rendered non-vital by previous trauma. Chipping of the incisal enamel in both central incisors is further evidence of trauma.

222

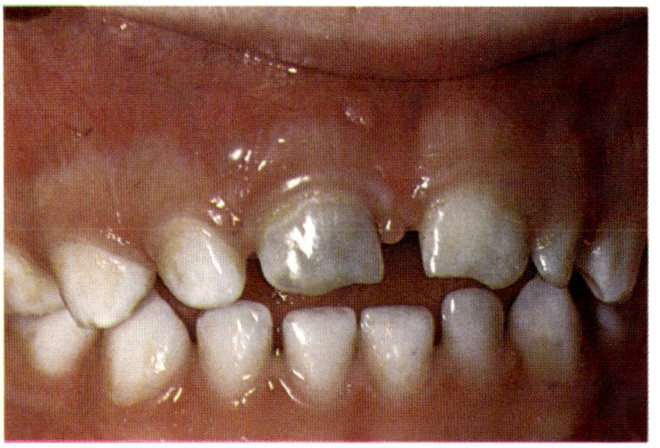

223 The radiograph of the incisor region seen in **222** shows root resorption of the right central incisor associated with periapical bony rarefaction.

223

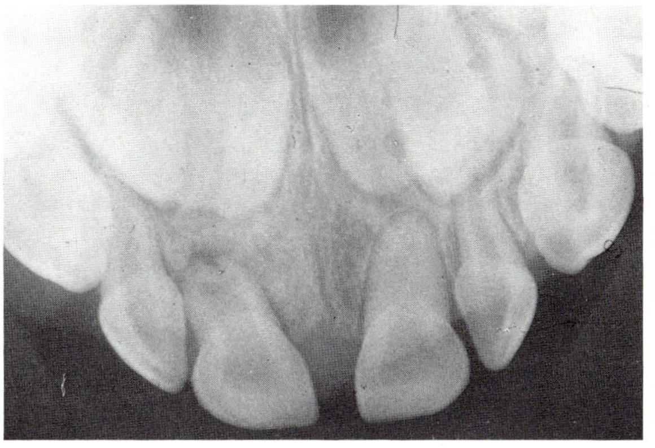

224 Pulpal calcification The partial calcific obliteration of the pulp chamber and root canal of the maxillary right central incisor was the result of a blow. The tooth became darker in colour, although it remained vital.

224

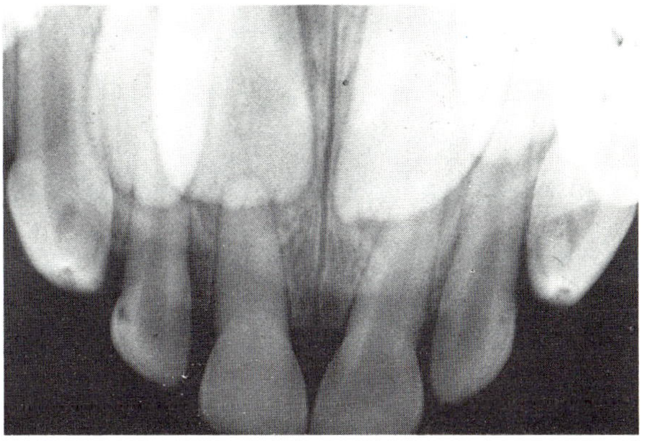

225 Avulsion This 18 month old child fell and avulsed the right maxillary canine from its socket. The tooth remains attached by only a few periodontal fibres on the palatal aspect.

225

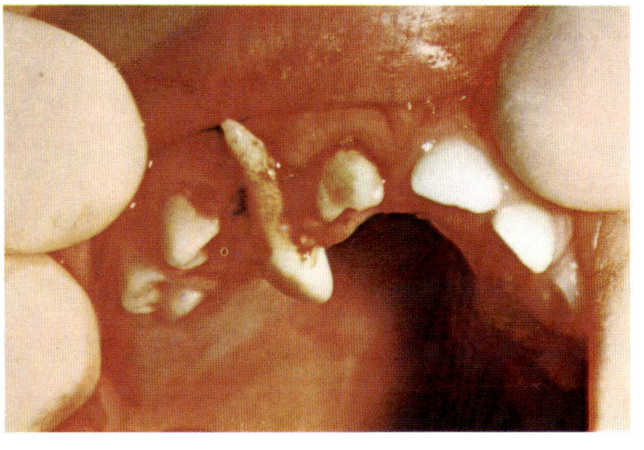

226

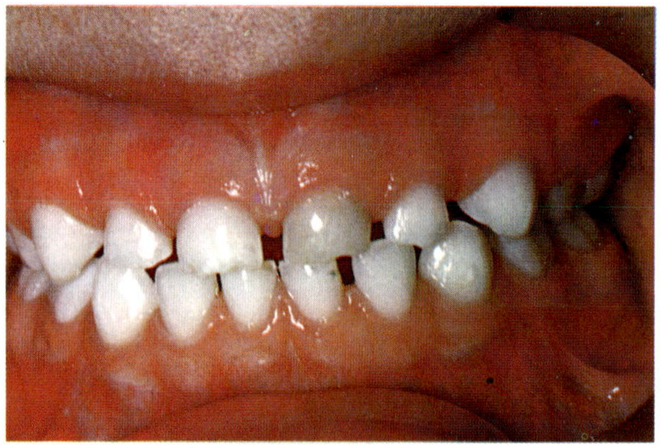

226 Coronal discolouration The faint coronal discolouration of the maxillary left central incisor is associated with a root canal filling.

227

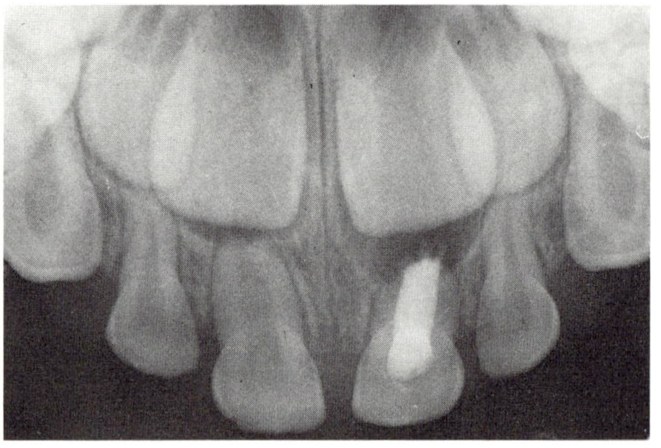

227 Radiograph of the incisor region showing a root canal filling of the maxillary left central incisor seen in **226**.

228

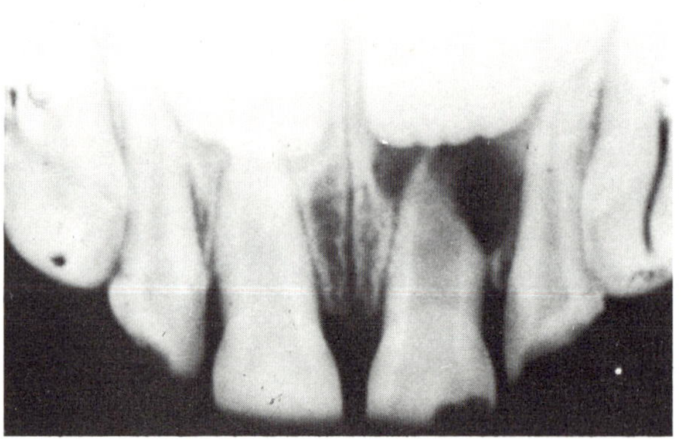

228 Coronal fracture with pulpal exposure A radiograph of the maxillary incisor region indicates an oblique coronal fracture of the left central incisor with pulpal exposure. It also shows evidence of abnormal root resorption and an area of periapical bony rarefaction which suggests chronic dentoalveolar infection.

229

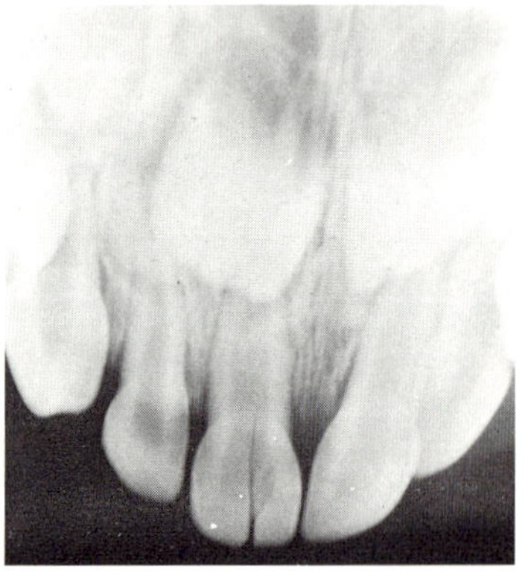

229 Fracture involving crown and root Trauma to the right maxillary central incisor has resulted in this unusual longitudinal fracture through the crown and root.

230 Root fracture A fall on to a concrete post caused the horizontal root fracture of the maxillary right central incisor.

230

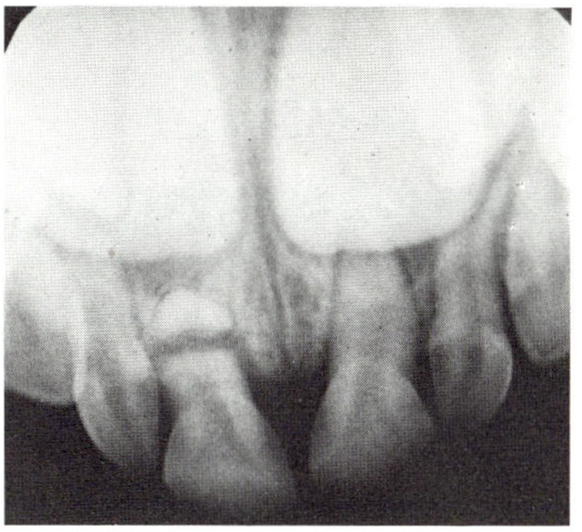

231 Intrusion A young child fell out of a high chair and intruded the maxillary right central incisor and completely avulsed the left central incisor from its socket. This radiograph shows the close relationship of the intruded incisor root to the overlying partially formed permanent central incisor and the fracture of the labial alveolar plate in the adjacent socket.

231

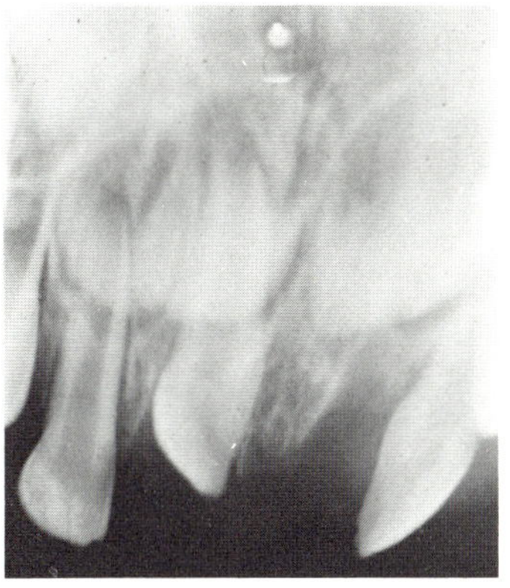

232 Dilaceration and hypoplasia Radiograph of a dilacerated and hypoplastic crown of the right maxillary permanent central incisor. A history of early trauma to the upper primary incisors was obtained from the parents.

232

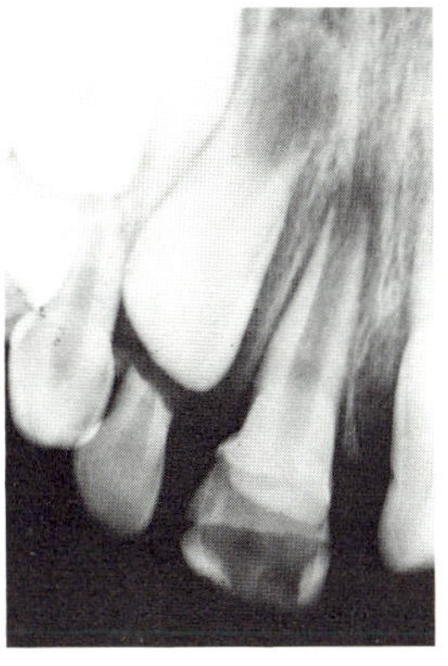

233 Sequestration of non-vital tooth The previously traumatised and non-vital maxillary right central incisor is in the process of sequestrating from the alveolus.

233

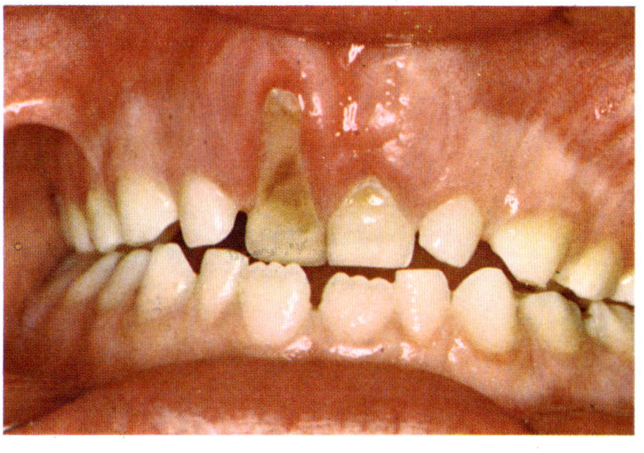

(ii) Permanent dentition

234

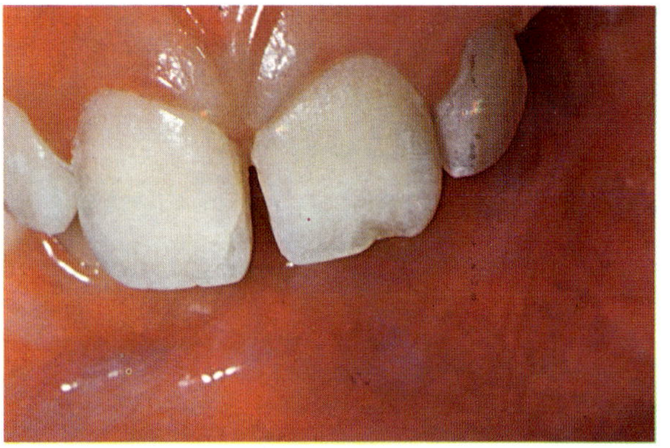

234 Coronal fracture – enamel Chipping of the enamel from the incisal edge of the maxillary left central incisor is the result of previous trauma. Note the crack in the enamel affecting the right central incisor.

235

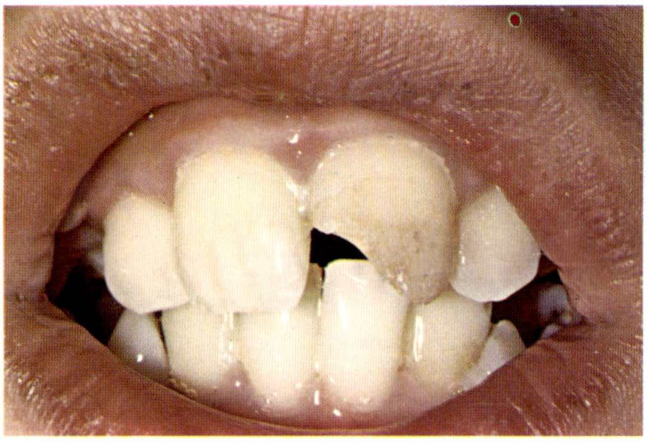

235 Coronal fracture – enamel and dentine Trauma to the maxillary left central incisor resulted in an oblique coronal fracture through the enamel and dentine. The pulp is not involved. Discolouration of the crown is the result of extrinsic staining of the exposed dentine.

236

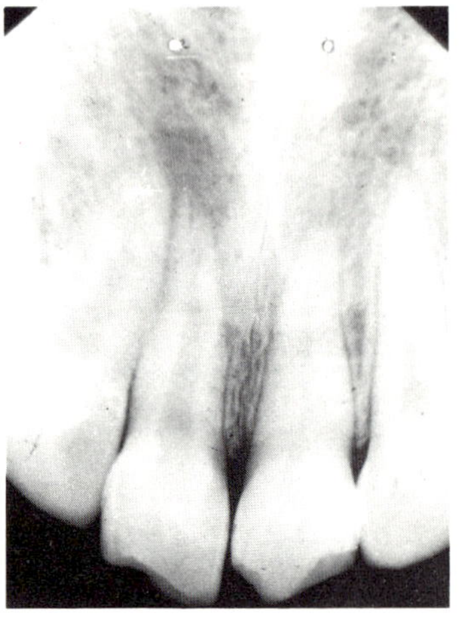

236 Coronal fracture – enamel and dentine This radiograph illustrates the occasional consequence of coronal trauma involving enamel and dentine (although the same may be seen with fractures of the enamel only). The periapical area of rarefaction associated with the fractured right central incisor is the result of a non-vital and infected pulp. Calcification of the pulp space in the fractured left central incisor indicates degenerative changes in the pulp subsequent to injury.

237, 238 Coronal fracture – enamel, dentine and pulp Severe trauma from a bicycle accident resulted in the coronal fracture of many incisor teeth. Frank pulpal exposure is evident in the maxillary right central incisor, and haemorrhage from the gingival margins around the left incisors suggests the possibility of the periodontal attachment of these teeth having been torn by a subluxation injury.

237

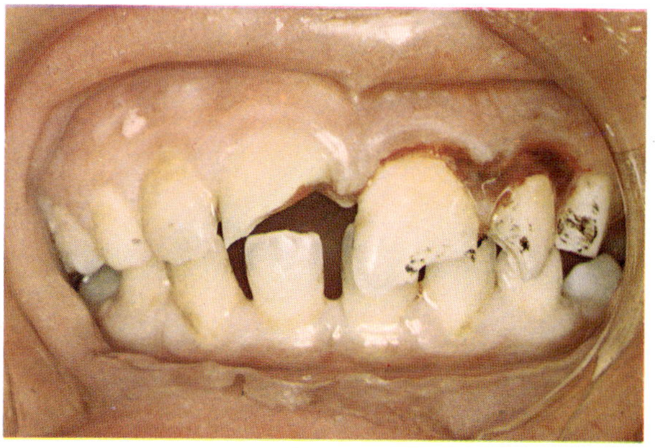

238

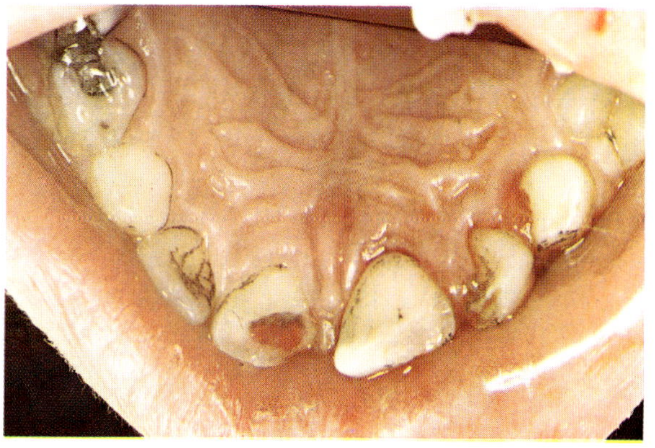

239 Root fracture Both maxillary central incisors have sustained horizontal fractures through the middle third of their roots.

239

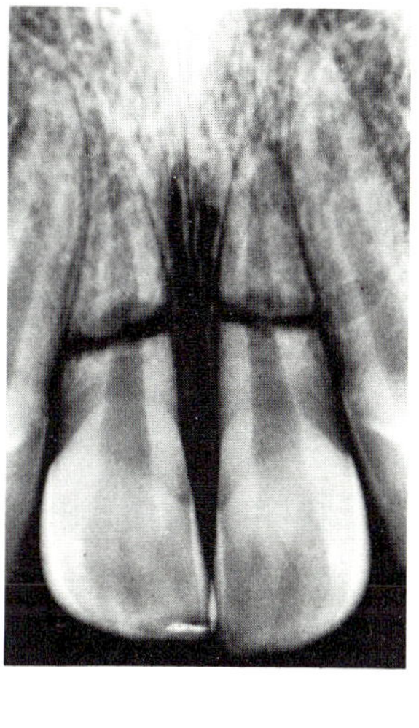

240

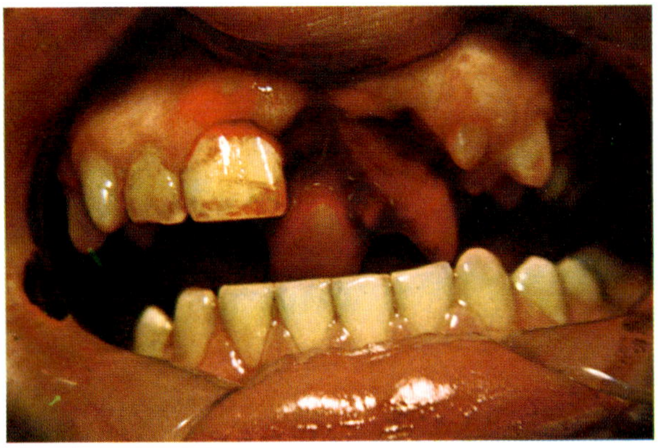

240 Avulsion The maxillary left incisors in this 15 year old boy were avulsed by a blow from a fist. The teeth were retained in the mouth by only a few periodontal fibres.

241

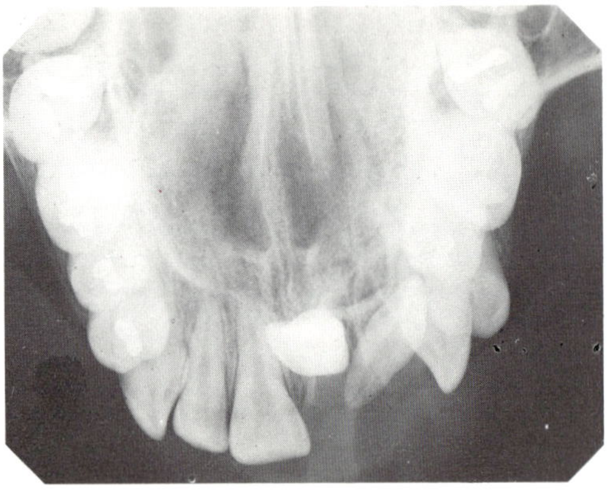

241 Radiograph of the condition shown in **240**.

242

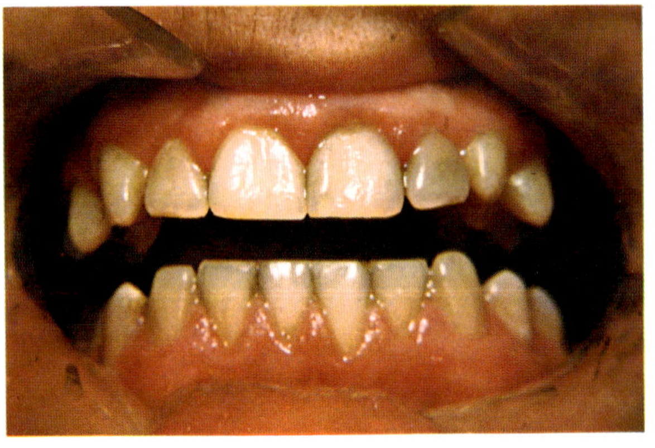

242 The maxillary left incisors shown in **240** were reimplanted in their sockets within the hour, splinted in place and subsequently root filled through the crown. Complete periodontal reattachment occurred but the crown of the lateral incisor discoloured slightly.

243

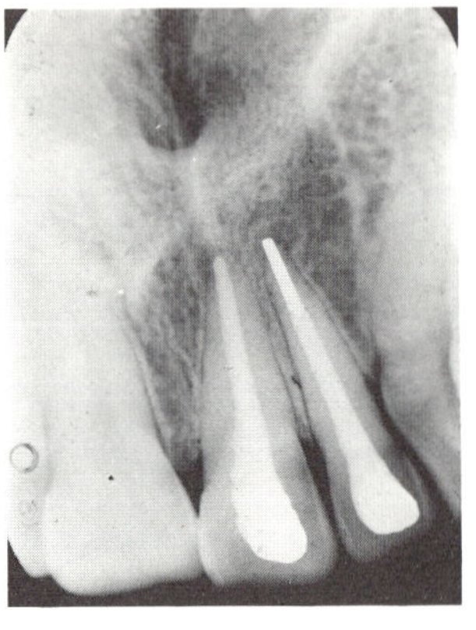

243 Radiograph of the incisors seen in **242** showing the appearance of the teeth subsequent to reattachment and root filling. Only minimal apical root resorption has occurred.

244 Root resorption The maxillary right central incisor had been avulsed five years previously, root filled and reimplanted in the socket. An acrylic splint was provided for fixation. Advanced root resorption is now evident around the root filling material.

244

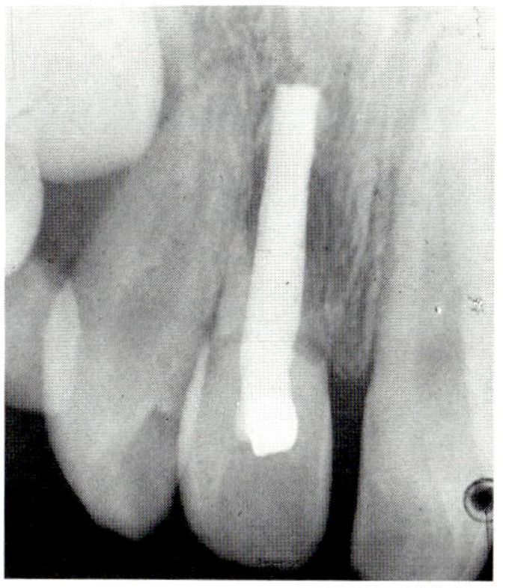

h. Caries

(i) Primary dentition

245, 246, 247 Rampant caries (Nursing bottle caries) The widespread rampant carious lesions in this 3 year old affected all the teeth except the lower six anteriors. The condition was associated with the use of a sweetened feeding bottle to comfort the child during the day and night. The dark staining of many of the affected teeth indicates a partial arrest of the condition. Note the chronic abscess pointing on to the mucogingival junction over the left maxillary canine in **245**.

245

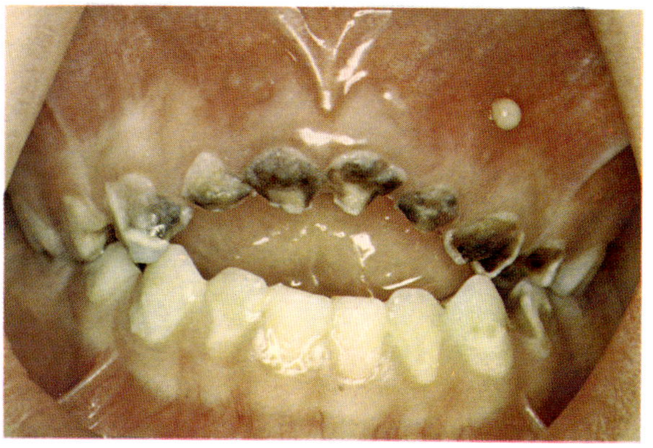

246

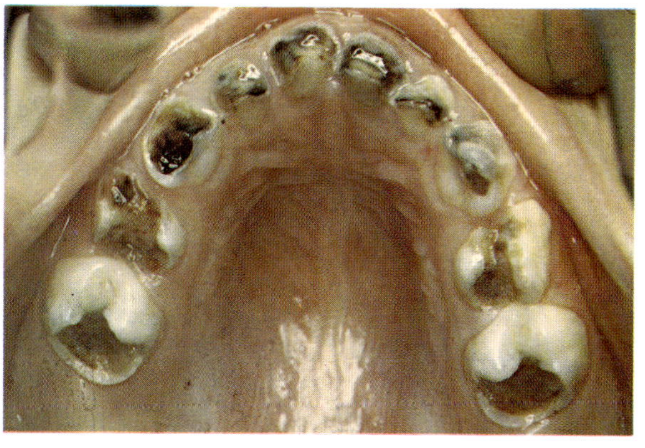

247

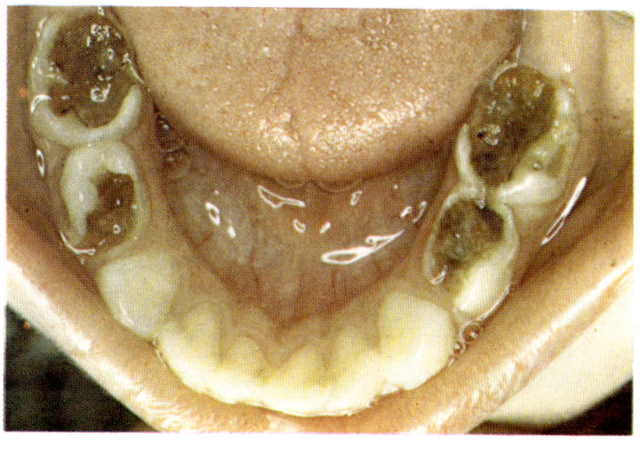

248 Arrested rampant caries The dark brown discolouration of the grossly decayed mandibular teeth in this 5 year old is associated with an arrest of the carious lesions. The surfaces of the carious dentine are all firm and the pulps are not exposed.

248

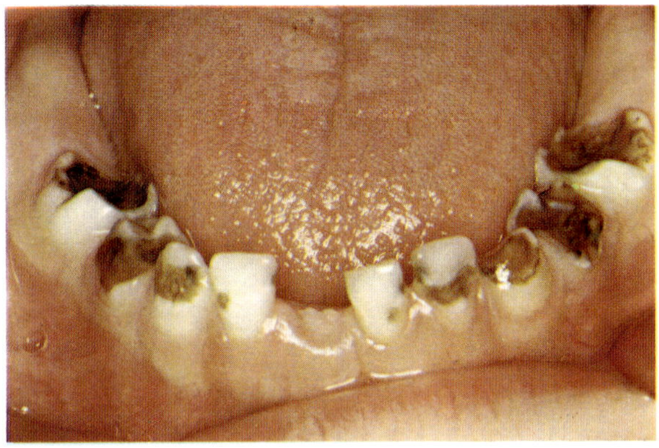

249 Rampant caries (Nursing bottle caries) The maxillary primary incisors and right canine of this 3 year old boy exhibit rampant carious lesions while the mandibular incisors remain caries-free. This common condition in young children is often the result of the child being provided with a feeding bottle containing a sweetened liquid or milk, for long periods, especially during sleeping hours. The tongue extends during swallowing to contact the lower lip, thereby covering the mandibular incisors and protecting them from the cariogenic effects of the ingested fluids.

249

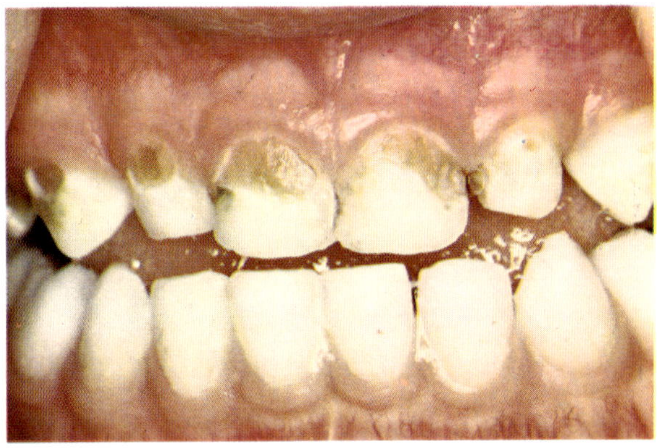

250 Arrested labial caries The brown stained linear defect on the labial surfaces of the maxillary incisors in this young child is evidence of arrest in early carious lesions. More active caries may be seen affecting the proximal surfaces of the central incisors. The linear defect is sometimes confused with neonatal enamel hypoplasia. The absence of enamel defects on the canines assists with the differential diagnosis.

250

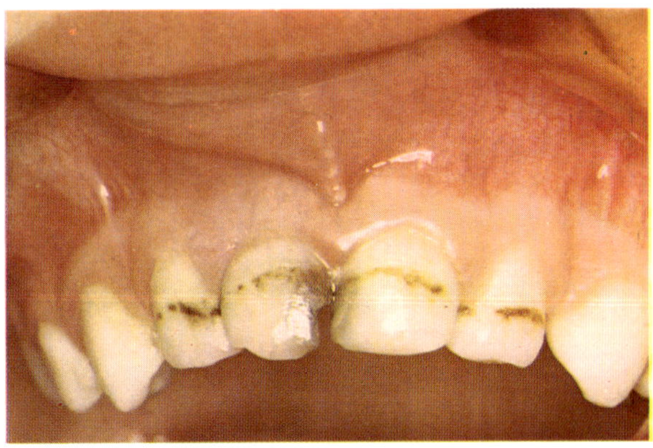

251 Occlusal caries Occlusal lesions in this young child affect all four molars in the mandible. The very large lesions in the first molars are associated with pulpal exposure.

251

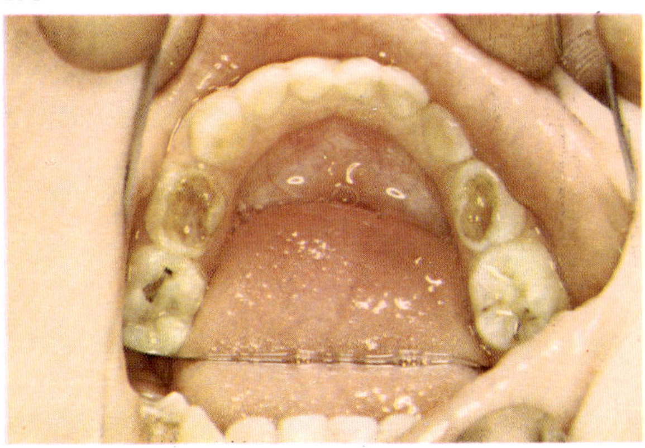

252, 253, 254 Progression of dental caries A series of bitewing radiographs from the same child showing the progression of proximal carious lesions affecting the distal surfaces of the first primary molars and the mesial surfaces of the second primary molars. With the breakdown of the marginal ridge on the distal aspect of the lower first molar and the close approximation of the carious lesion to the pulp, a possible pulpal exposure should be anticipated.

252

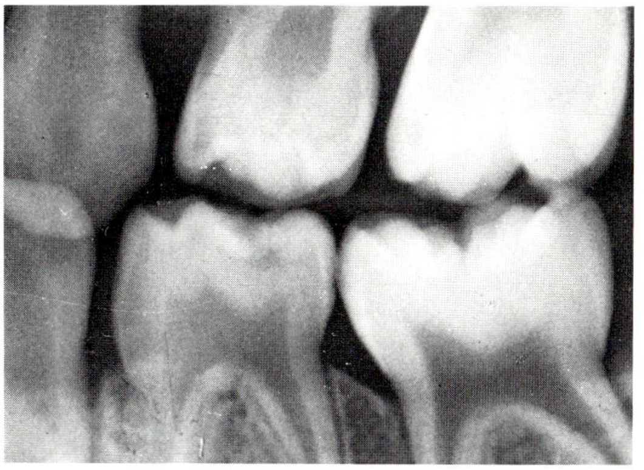

253

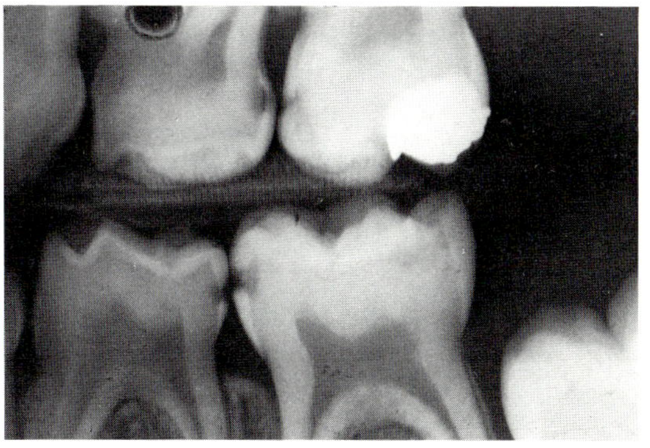

254

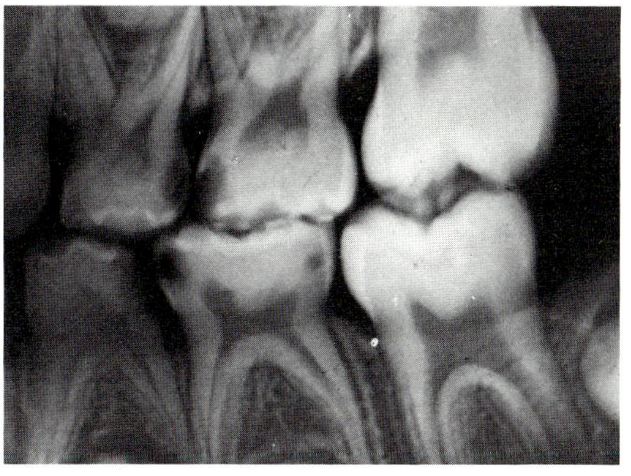

(ii) Permanent dentition

255 Lower incisor caries Proximal caries in the mandibular incisor teeth of teenagers, as seen in this patient, is a poor prognostic sign for the future of the dentition unless early control of the disease can be effected.

255

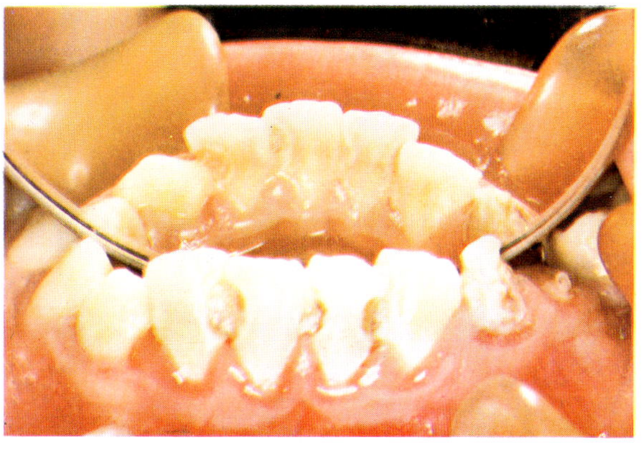

256 Malocclusion and caries Severe crowding of teeth makes plaque control difficult and is likely to be associated with proximal carious lesions. In this adolescent, such carious lesions are seen in both upper and lower incisor teeth.

256

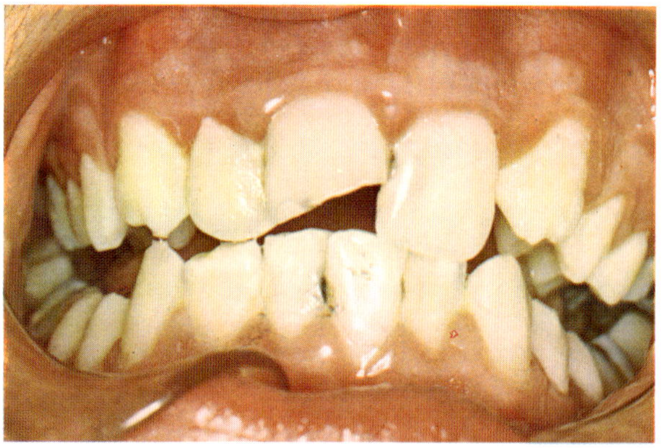

257 Orthodontic bands and caries The whitish cervical area of demineralisation on the buccal surface of the mandibular first permanent molar is an incipient carious lesion which followed the loss of dental cement from beneath an orthodontic band.

257

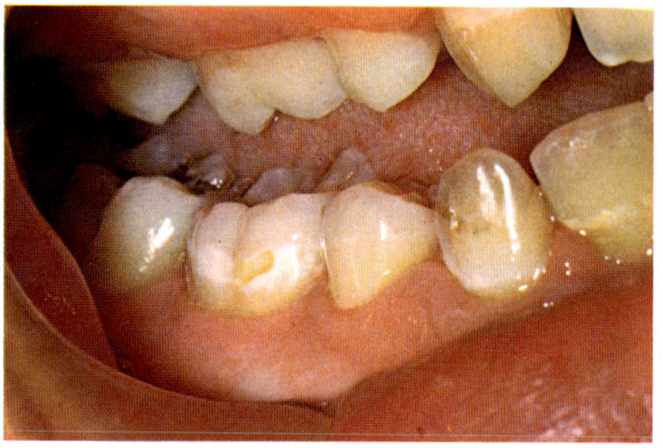

i. Pulp

258 Pulpal necrosis associated with caries Radiograph showing evidence of periapical and inter-radicular rarefaction affecting the mandibular first primary molar. The large distal carious lesion suggests the possibility of pulpal exposure with subsequent infection and necrosis of the pulpal tissues. Spread of infection to the periradicular tissues has resulted in bony destruction and abscess formation.

258

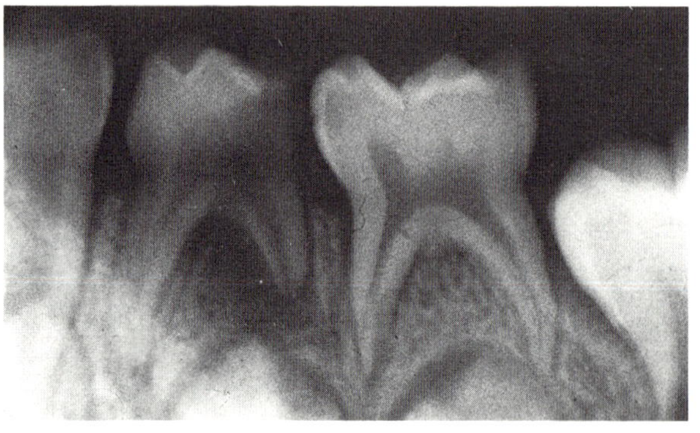

259 Pulpal necrosis associated with dens invaginatus This radiograph shows an invaginated maxillary right permanent lateral incisor with incomplete root formation (open apex) and a very large area of periapical bony rarefaction. Pulpal infection and necrosis are occasionally associated with the presence of such invaginations which are incompletely lined by enamel. The bony lesion in this case proved to be associated with apical cyst formation.

259

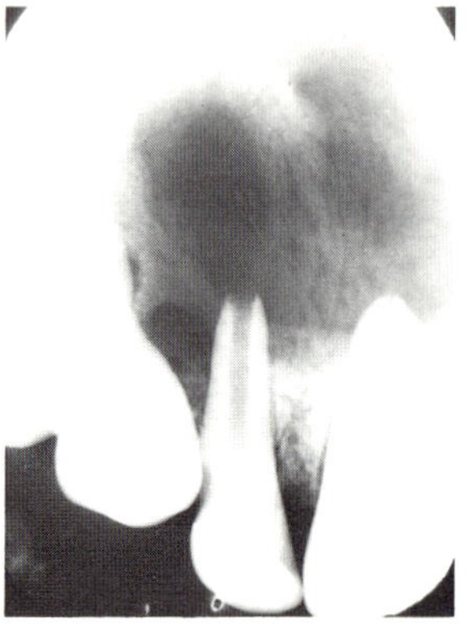

260 Chronic hyperplastic pulpitis An untreated exposed pulp in the traumatised maxillary permanent central incisor has been followed by chronic infection and the development of a hyperplastic pulpitis, as is evidenced by the bright red pulp polyp on the palatal aspect of the crown.

260

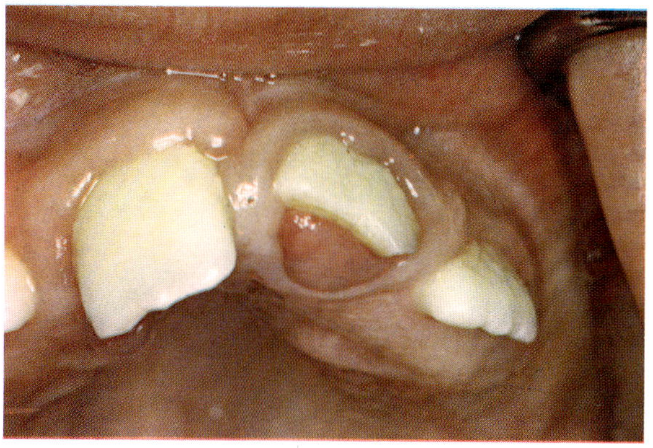

261 Chronic hyperplastic pulpitis A pulp polyp is growing out of the occlusal surface of the mandibular first permanent molar. The result of chronic hyperplastic pulpitis following carious destruction of the crown and pulpal exposure.

261

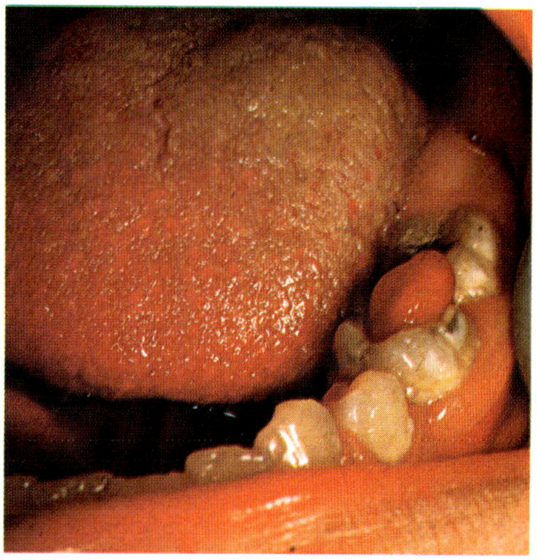

262 Internal resorption Resorption occurring within the pulp space of the maxillary right permanent central incisor has caused a perforation of the labial enamel and dentine in the cervical portion of the crown.

262

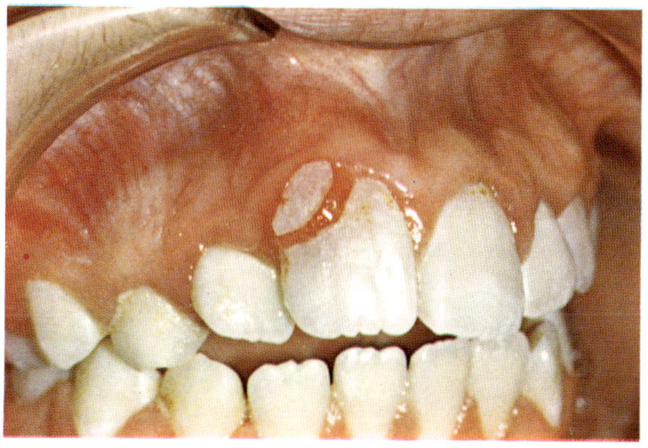

3. Gingival and periodontal conditions

a. Gingiva

263 Congenital epulis This newly born baby shows a pedunculated swelling attached to the gingival mucosa of the premaxilla. These congenital malformations are benign and do not recur after adequate local excision. Histologically the lesion resembles a granular cell myoblastoma but the cell of origin is uncertain.

263

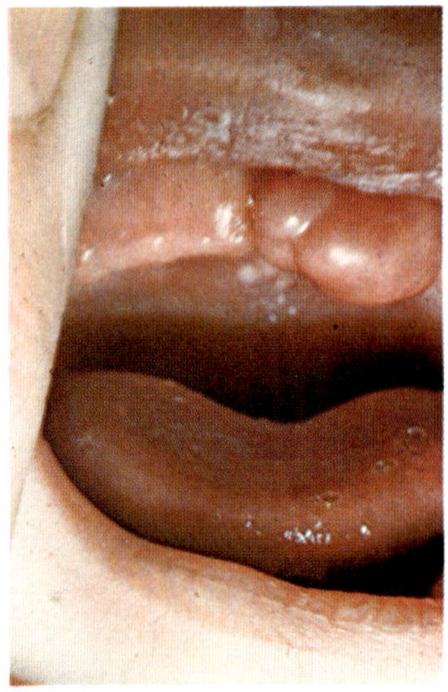

264 Gingival cyst (Bohn's nodule) The small whitish nodule in the gingival mucosa of the mandibular gum pad of this infant is known as a Bohn's nodule. It consists of a microcyst developed from epithelial remnants within the gingival tissues. These lesions are common in infancy and undergo spontaneous resolution a few months following birth.

264

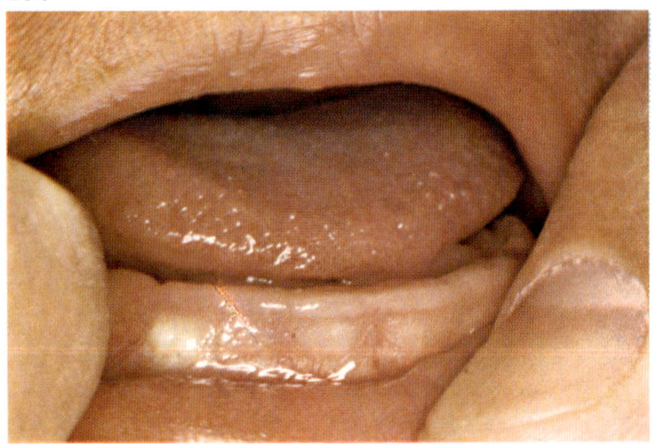

265 Eruption haematoma A bluish lesion appeared on the labial aspect of the maxillary gum pad over the site of an erupting primary central incisor in this infant. The lesion was opaque to transillumination and was due to haemorrhage into the tissues. Treatment was not required and the tooth erupted into the mouth several days later.

265

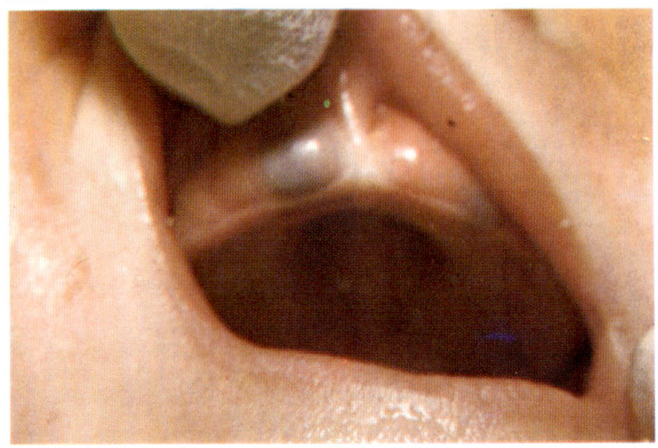

266 **Eruption cyst** The bluish swelling overlying the unerupted maxillary right central incisor in this 7 year old boy is typical of an eruption cyst. Excision biopsy of a portion of the overlying mucosa demonstrated a histological appearance consistent with a dentigerous or eruption cyst. While most eruption cysts are filled with clear fluid and transilluminate brilliantly, this one was filled with blood.

266

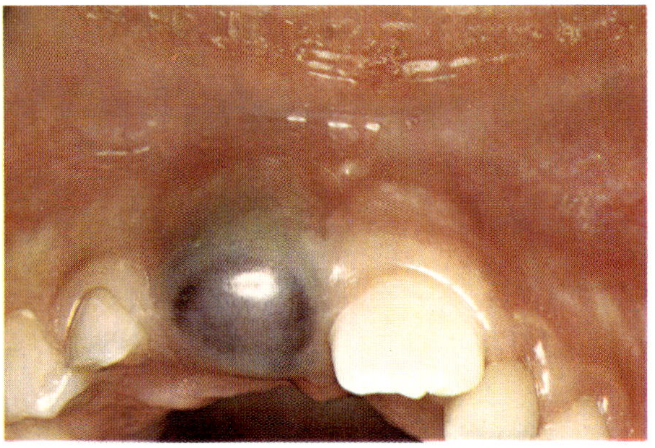

267 **Upper labial frenum** Although there is a wide diastema between the maxillary primary central incisors in this young child, the labial frenum is normal and does not require treatment.

267

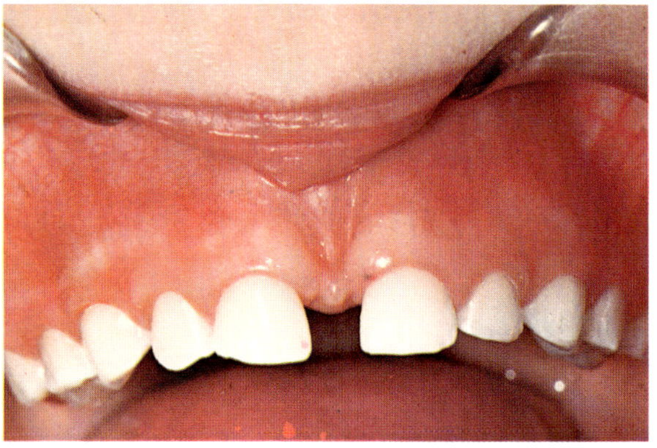

268 **Upper labial frenum** The large maxillary labial frenum in this 7 year old girl is associated with a midline diastema between the central incisors. A decision on frenectomy was postponed until the lateral incisors and canines had erupted.

268

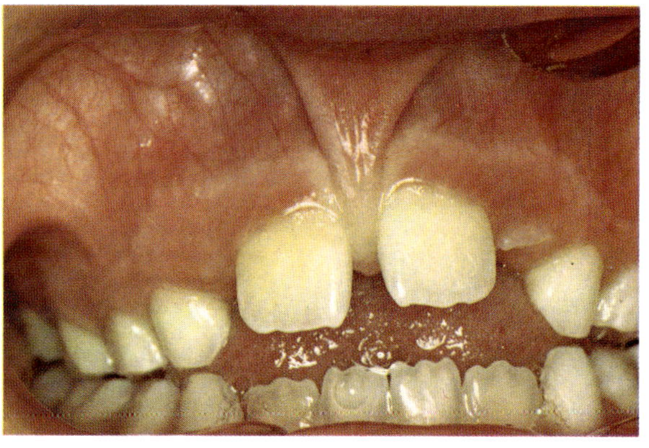

269 **Lower labial frenum** An abnormal attachment of the mandibular labial frenum into the gingival tissues adjacent to the primary central incisors is present in this 4 year old girl. Frena of this type are occasionally associated with localised gingival recession and should be kept under careful observation.

269

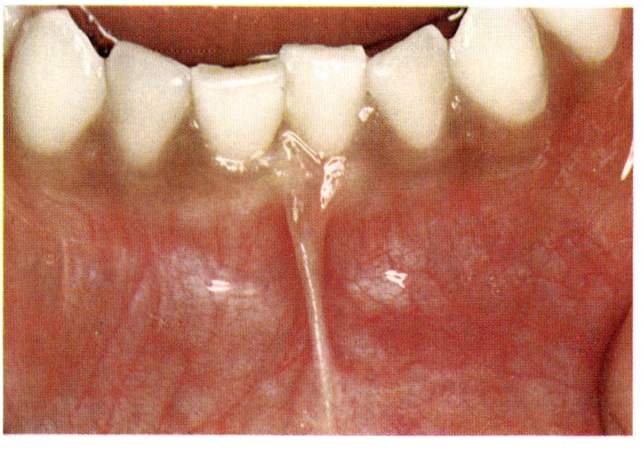

270 Localised gingival recession The exposed root surface of this supplemental mandibular incisor is associated with a localised form of gingival recession. Extraction of the supernumerary tooth resulted in complete resolution of the condition, which suggests that lower incisor crowding was the principal aetiological agent.

270

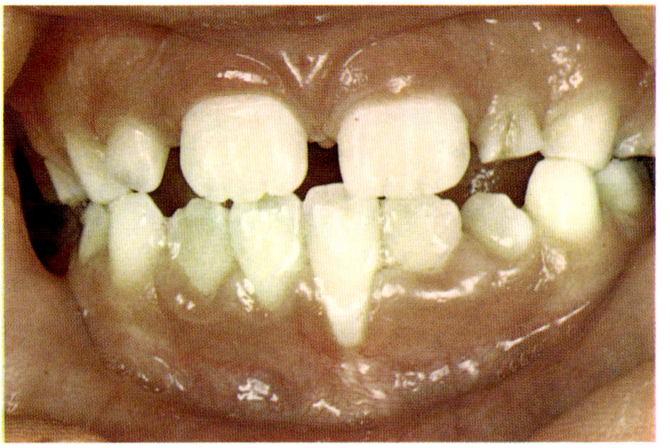

271 Localised gingival recession Bilateral gingival recession affecting both mandibular permanent central incisors is present in this 12 year old girl. Root surface is exposed on both teeth. The condition appeared to be associated with a cloth sucking habit at night. An orthodontic appliance was used to help her stop the habit. Once the habit ceased the gingival condition remained static.

271

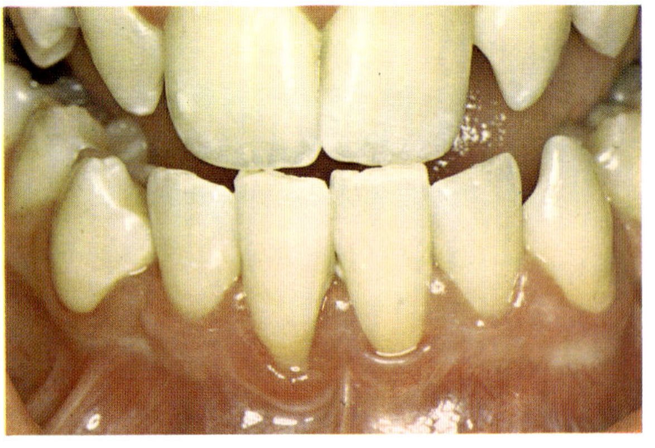

272 Localised gingival recession This 3 year old boy presented with gingival recession affecting the labial aspects of all the mandibular primary incisors. He had been sucking a dummy (pacifier), with the plastic rim held inside his lower lip, for more than two years.

272

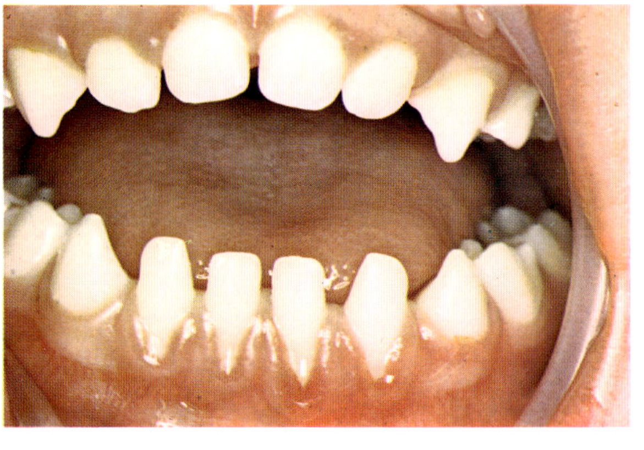

273

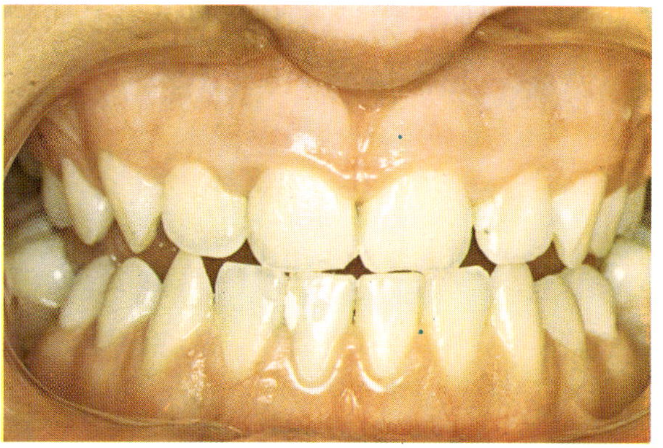

273 Delayed gingival retreat (Retarded passive eruption) The clinical crowns of the upper incisor teeth in this 11 year old girl remained small due to failure of the gingiva to recede towards the amelo-cemental junction. The gingival sulcus was abnormally deep and the child was unable to remove plaque from these sites with resultant chronic marginal gingivitis.

274

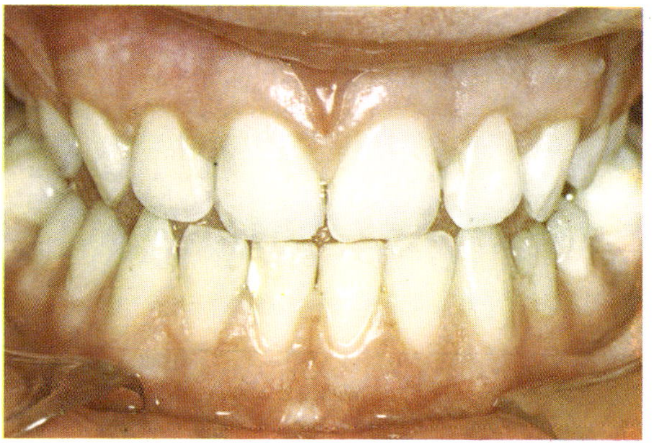

274 Recontour of the gingiva shown in **273** under local anaesthesia improved aesthetics and enabled the upper incisors to be kept free of plaque.

275

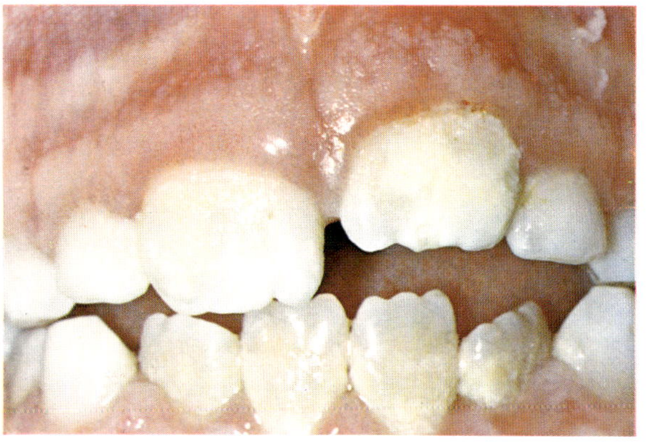

275 Dental plaque A heavy deposition of plaque and other debris on the incisors of this patient with a mixed dentition who neglected proper oral hygiene procedures.

276

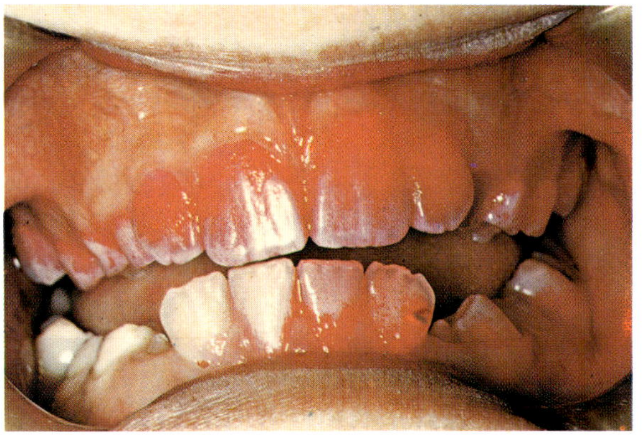

276 Identification of plaque A disclosing solution has stained the dental plaque coating the teeth of this child with periodontitis.

277

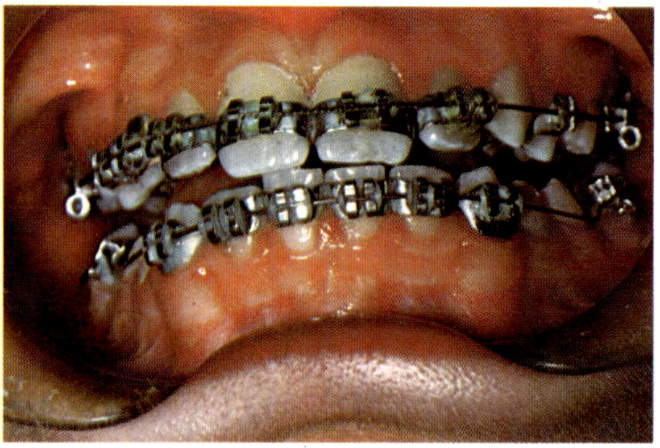

277 Chronic marginal gingivitis A mild gingivitis in a teenager wearing an orthodontic appliance.

278

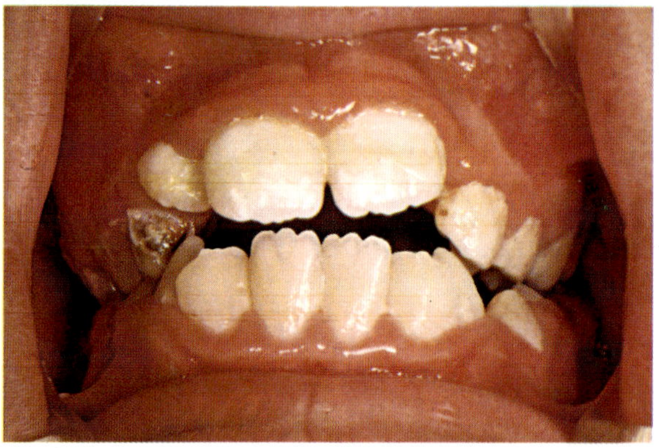

278 Chronic marginal gingivitis The gingivae of a healthy child in the mixed dentition stage of occlusal development. As the result of poor oral hygiene there is a moderate degree of chronic marginal gingivitis.

279

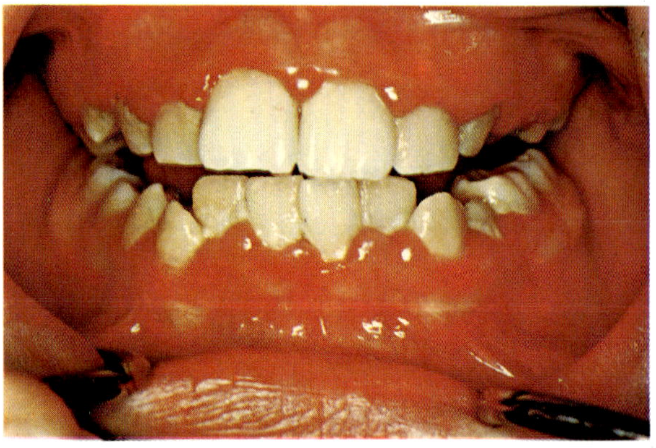

279 Chronic marginal gingivitis This child illustrates a more severe form of gingivitis due to inadequate oral hygiene procedures.

280

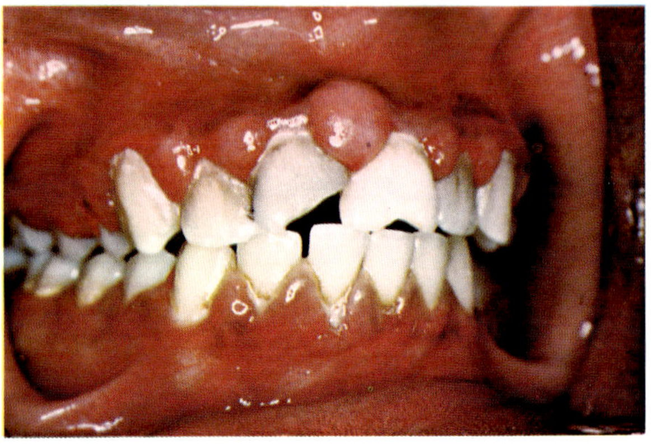

280 Chronic hyperplastic gingivitis Marked gingival hyperplasia in response to chronic gingivitis in a pubescent patient with an untreated malocclusion and very poor oral hygiene.

281 Chronic hyperplastic gingivitis Poor oral hygiene combined with incisal crowding in this pregnant teenage girl is responsible for the chronic hyperplastic gingivitis which is most marked in the lower incisor region.

281

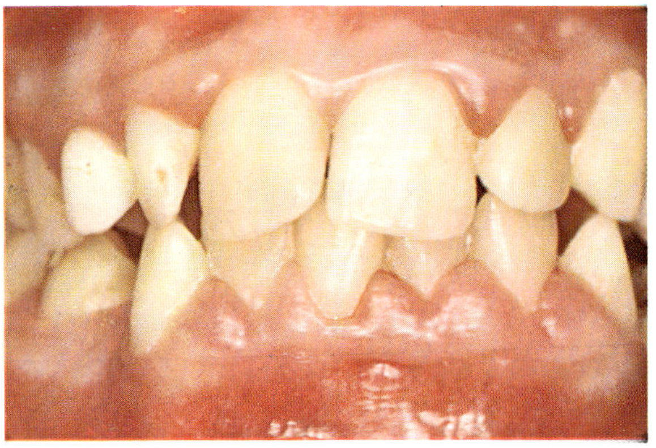

282 Puberty gingivitis Plaque and stain on the incisor teeth of this pubescent girl indicate the neglect of oral hygiene procedures which has given rise to the chronic marginal gingivitis. The exaggerated inflammatory response seen in some females during puberty is thought to be hormonal in origin.

282

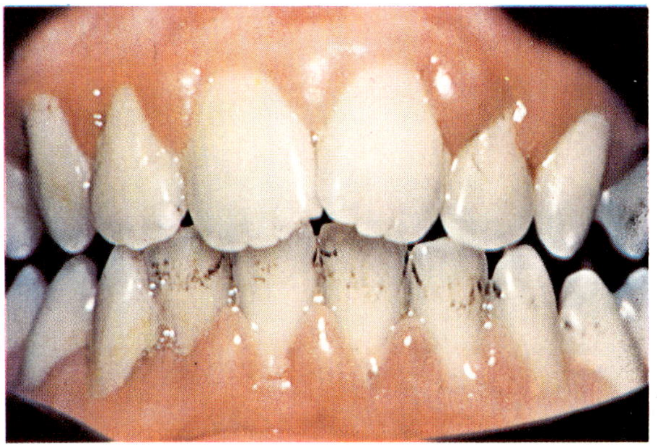

283 Acute necrotising ulcerative gingivitis (Vincent's infection) Considerable pain and bleeding accompanied the destructive gingival ulceration in this 15 year old girl with Vincent's infection. Characteristically the interdental papillae show the greatest changes. The diagnosis was confirmed by bacterial smear and culture.

283

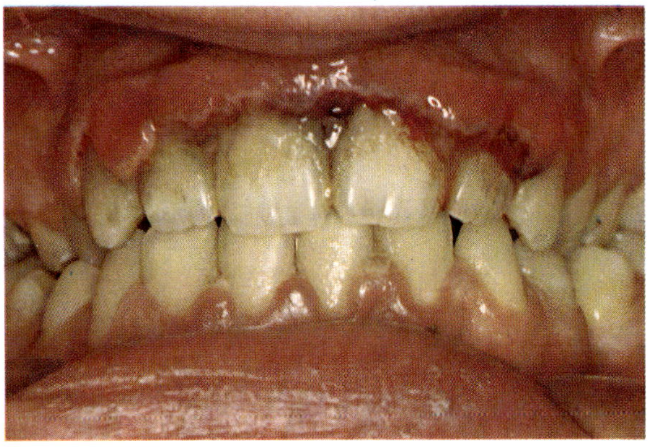

284 Phenytoin gingival hyperplasia The gingival hyperplasia affecting this epileptic child treated with phenytoin sodium (Dilantin, Epanutin) is commonly seen in such patients. The gross enlargement of the interdental papillae is particularly characteristic of the condition.

284

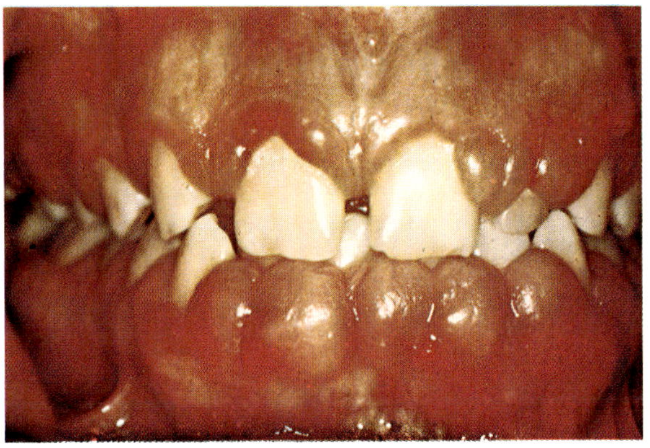

285, 286 **Hereditary gingival hyperplasia** The gross thickening of the gingivae was present in this girl at 7 years in the primary dentition and at 13 years with the eruption of the permanent teeth. Gingival enlargement was noted from infancy and was associated with hypertrichosis. Delayed eruption of teeth was a feature in both dentitions and the abnormal eruption of maxillary permanent incisors may be seen. The usual mode of genetic transmission for this anomaly is by an autosomal dominant gene. (See **470**)

285

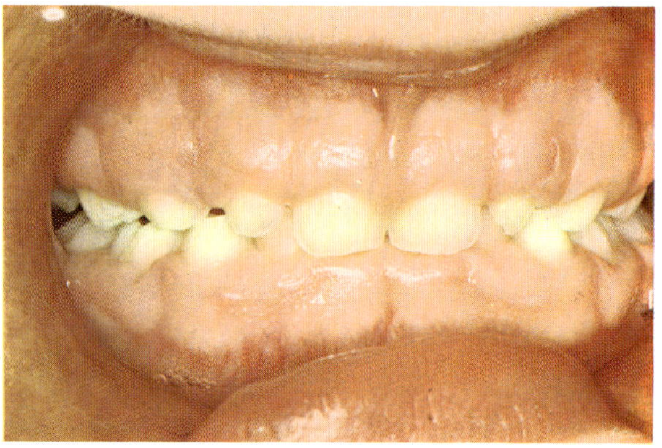

286

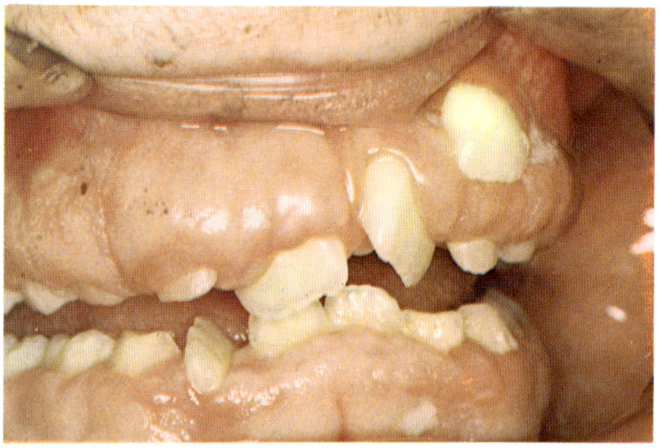

287 Localised gingival hyperplasia Histologically the localised gingival enlargement in the maxillary incisor region of this child is identical to that seen in hereditary gingival hyperplasia.

287

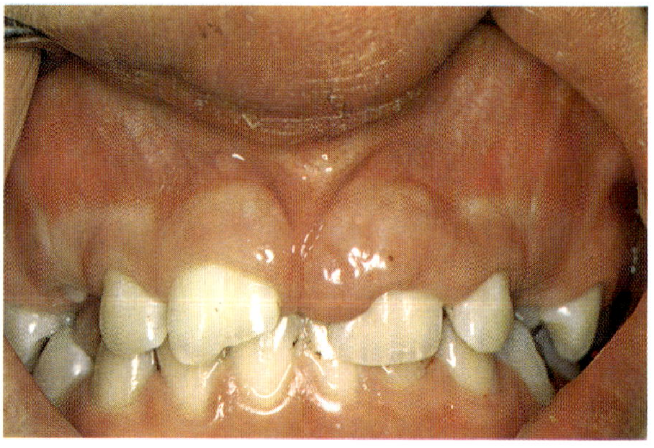

288 Acute herpetic gingivostomatitis Marked gingival redness and swelling is evident in the lower molar region of this 6 year old child with acute herpetic gingivostomatitis. The intact vesicle on the mucosa of the lower lip is typical of viral infections of this type and requires differentiation from varicella and Coxsackie virus infections.

288

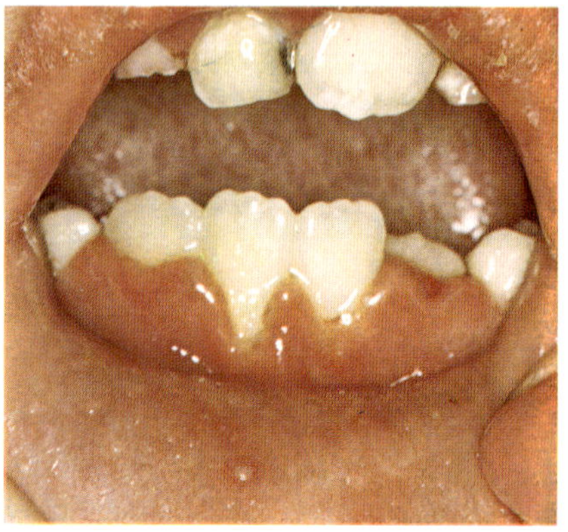

289 Herpes zoster The gingival ulceration in this 17 year old boy was noted during an acute attack of herpes zoster. (See **40** and **389**)

289

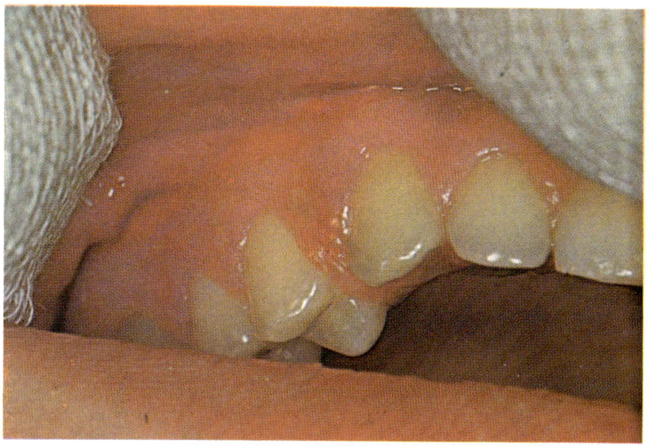

290 Desquamative gingivitis The intense redness of the gingivae in this teenage girl is associated with a superficial desquamation of the gingival epithelium. Despite the generalised and chronic nature of this condition, the patient appeared to suffer relatively little discomfort. The cause is unknown.

290

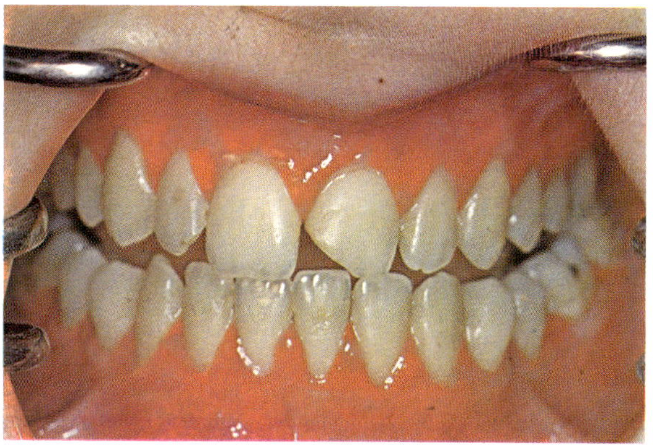

291 Desquamative gingivitis The gingivitis present in the lower incisor region of this teenager exhibited a desquamation of the superficial layers of the epithelium. A history of psoriasis was obtained.

291

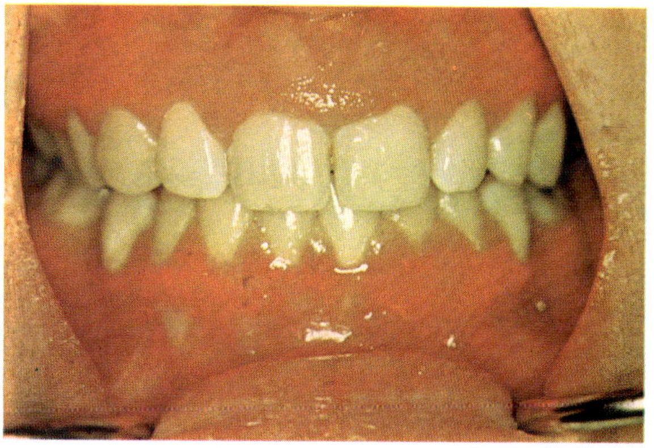

292 Desquamative gingivitis A desquamative gingivitis localised to the incisor region of this 9 year old boy was present for several years and failed to respond to treatment. Recurrent aphthous ulceration was also noted in this patient.

292

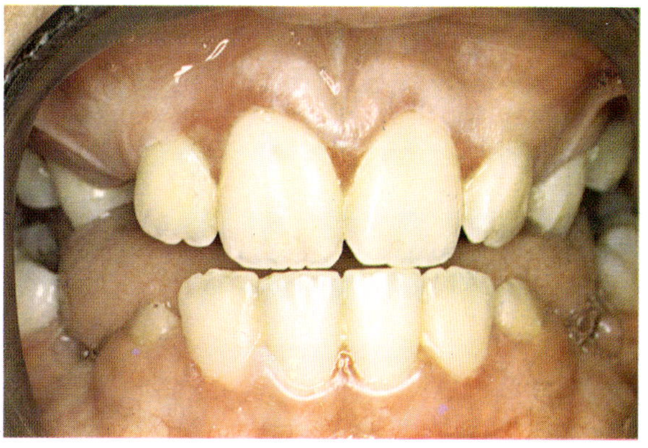

293

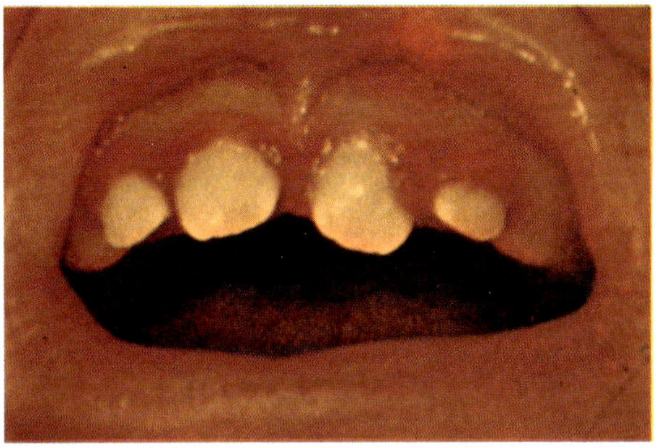

293 Scorbutic gingivitis This 14 month old infant with scurvy from prolonged vitamin C deficiency shows an intense inflammatory redness of the gingiva around the maxillary incisors.

294

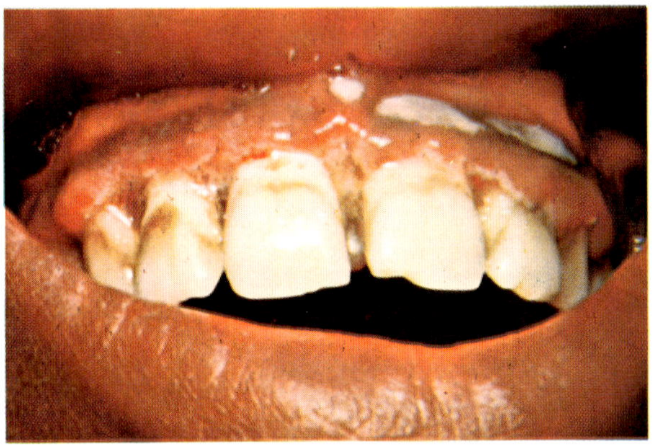

294 Infectious mononucleosis A marked gingivitis with ulceration of the gingival margins is present in this teenager in the advanced stages of infectious mononucleosis.

295

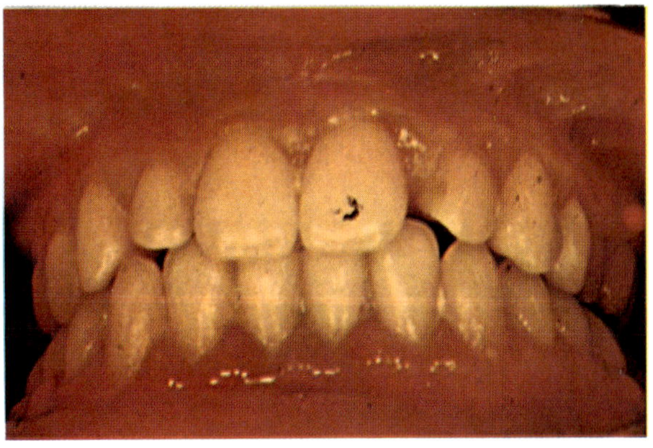

295 Juvenile diabetes Inflammatory changes in the gingival tissues are most marked in the lower incisor region of this patient with diabetes mellitus.

296

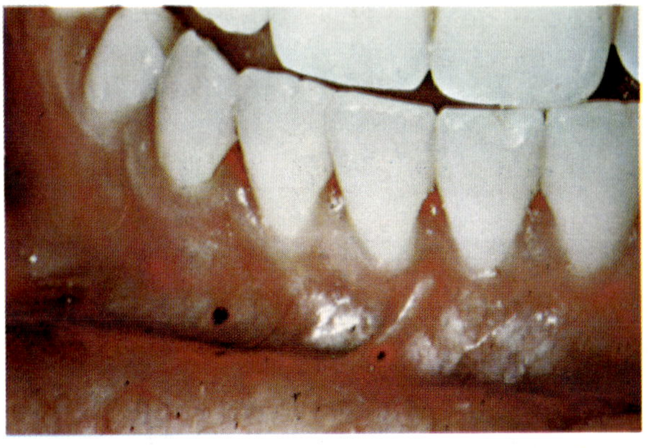

296 Aplastic anaemia Spontaneous bleeding from the interdental papillae and petechial haemorrhages into the alveolar mucosa are seen in this child with aplastic anaemia. Extreme pallor of the mucous membranes is another feature of this condition.

297 Periodic (Cyclic) neutropenia A persistent chronic gingivitis remains present in this child with periodic neutropenia despite repeated prophylaxis and careful attention to oral hygiene procedures. (See **420**)

297

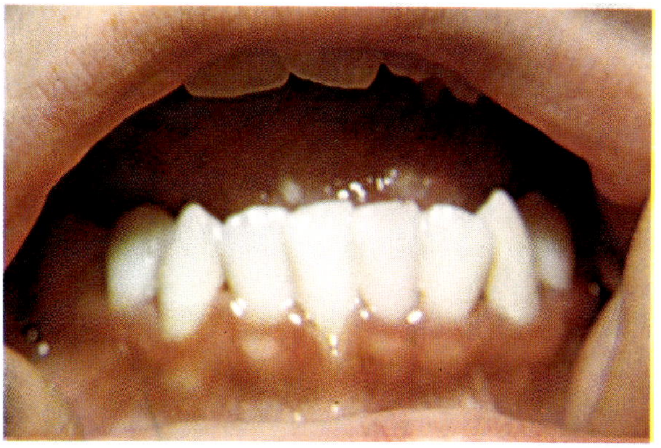

298 Thrombocytopenia Spontaneous bleeding from the gingival margins was a marked feature in this adolescent with generalised purpura associated with essential (primary) thrombocytopenia. The condition resolved after splenectomy. (See **471**)

298

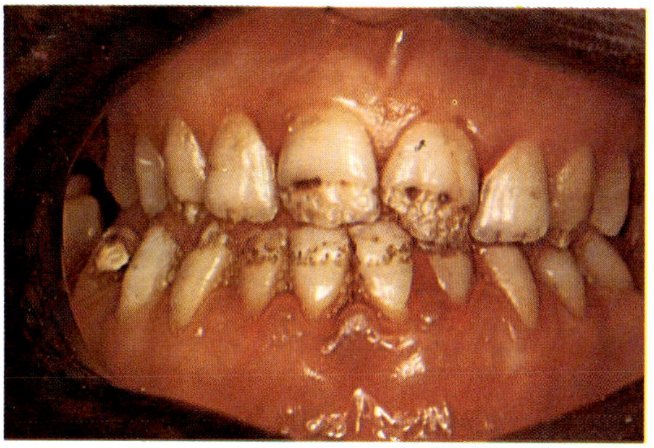

299 Actinomycosis Gingival ulceration and swelling are present buccal to the mandibular right first primary molar in this 8 year old child.

299

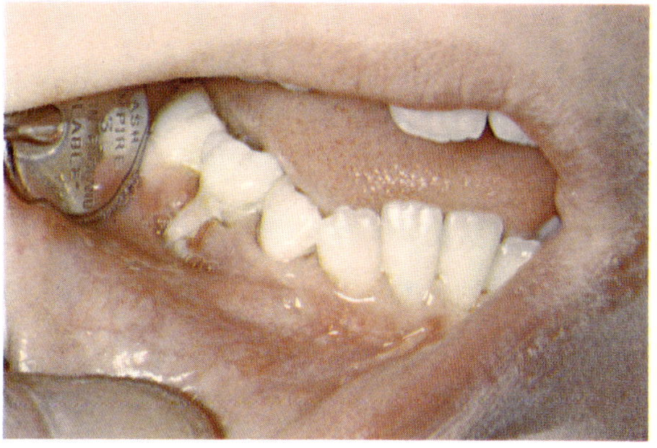

300 Racial gingival pigmentation The dark brown pigmentation of the gingiva in this teenager is due to the physiological deposition of melanin within the tissues and is a racial characteristic.

300

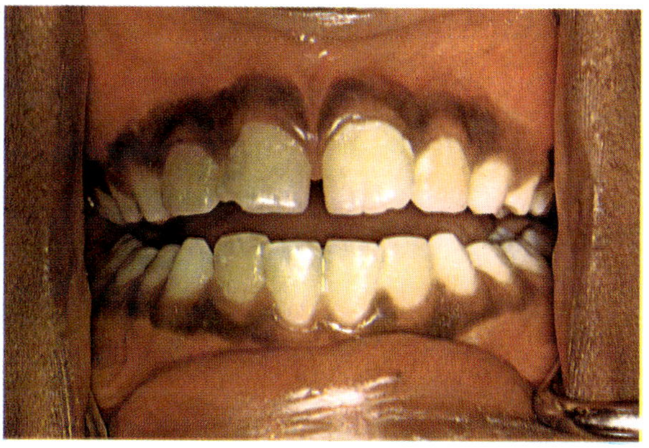

301

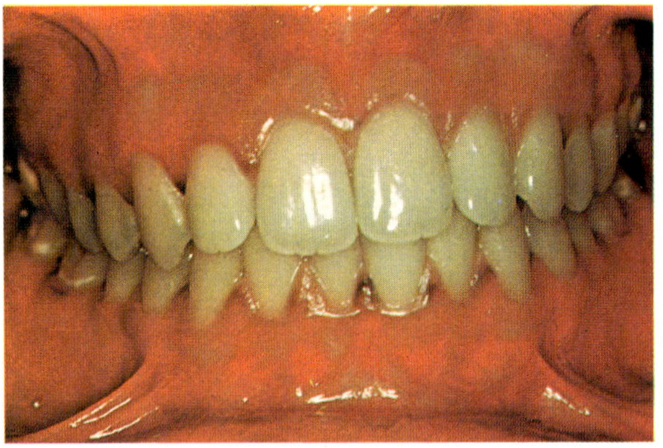

301 Addison's disease Many of the interdental papillae in this adolescent with adrenal cortical insufficiency are pigmented a dark brown colour due to the pathological deposition of melanin within the tissues.

302

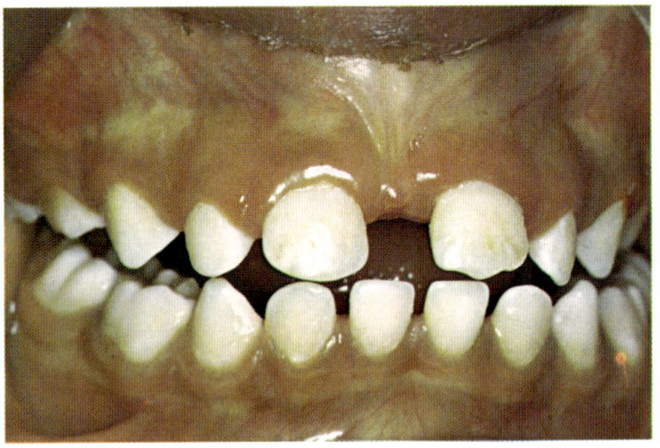

302 Sickle cell anaemia This 4 year old girl with severe sickle cell anaemia is persistently jaundiced. The gingival tissues are stained yellow by the deposition of excessive amounts of bile pigment. (See **55**)

303

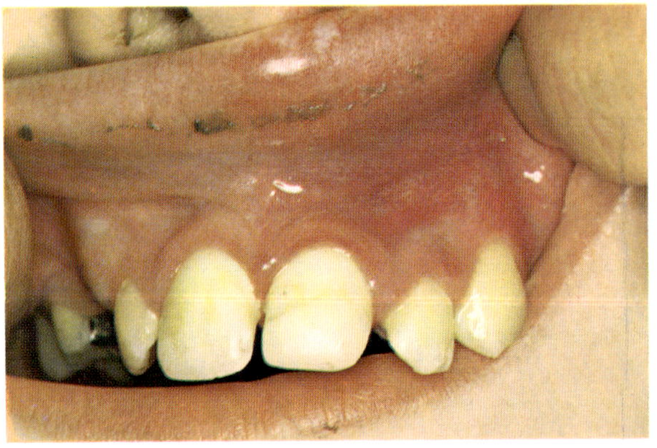

303 Capillary haemangioma Bright red discolouration of gingiva and alveolar mucosa on the left side of the maxilla is due to the presence of a capillary haemangioma. (See **26**)

304

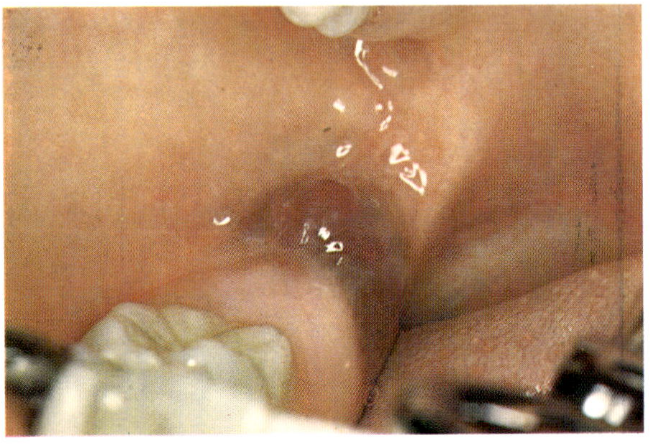

304 Cavernous haemangioma The localised bluish-red swelling of the gum pad disto-lingual to the mandibular right second permanent molar was caused by the presence of a cavernous haemangioma. The lesion was removed by cryosurgery.

305

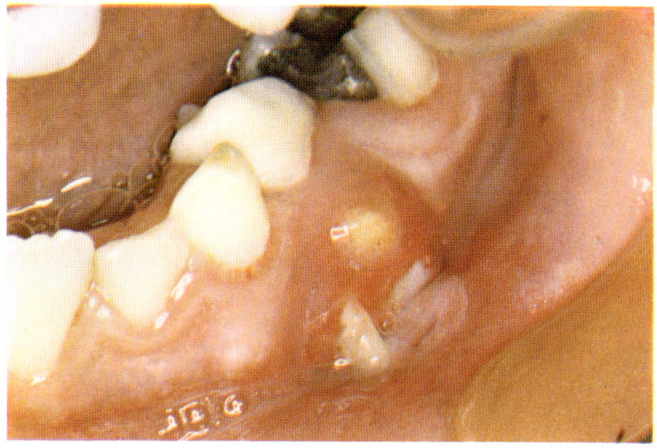

305 Chronic dentoalveolar abscess (Gum boil) The localised yellowish swelling of the attached gingiva buccal to the first primary molar is associated with a chronic dentoalveolar abscess derived from the adjacent cariously exposed, non-vital and infected tooth.

306

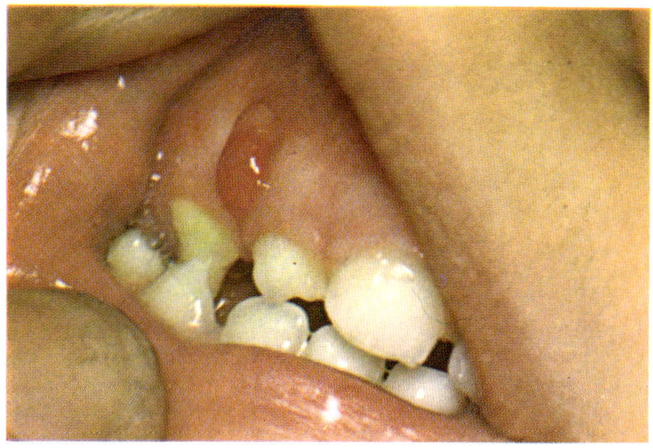

306 Granulation tissue The swelling overlying the maxillary primary lateral incisor is due to the proliferation of granulation tissue from an apical sinus. The chipped enamel on the incisor is evidence of previous trauma and suggests the possibility of a non-vital and infected tooth as the cause of the condition.

307

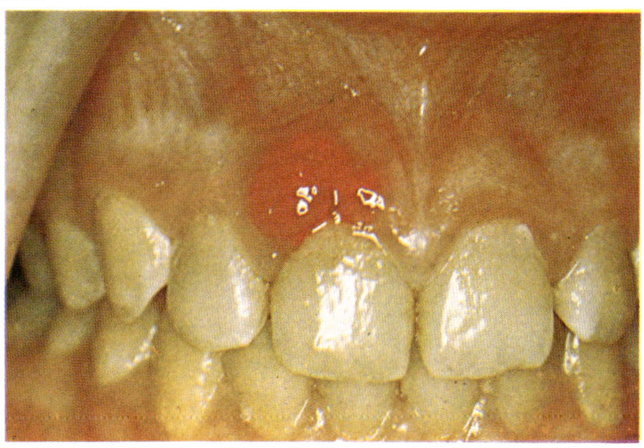

307 Granulation tissue Following trauma to the gingival tissues in the maxillary incisor region, this sessile mass of reddish granulation tissue was noted.

308

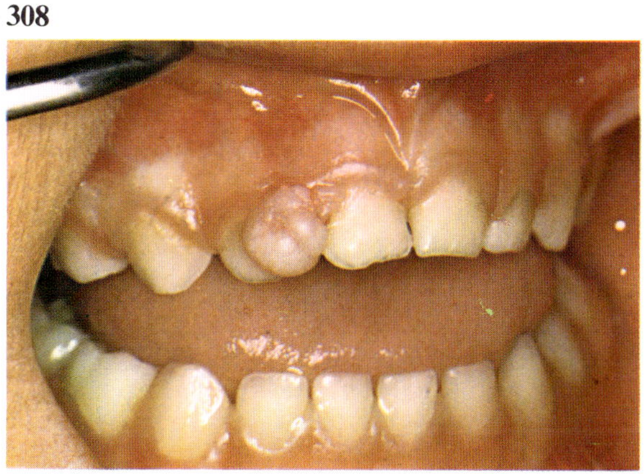

308 Fibroepithelial polyp (Giant cell fibroma) The pedunculated swelling on the gingiva overlying the maxillary primary lateral incisor had been present for 10 weeks. Excision biopsy showed it to be a fibroepithelial polyp.

309

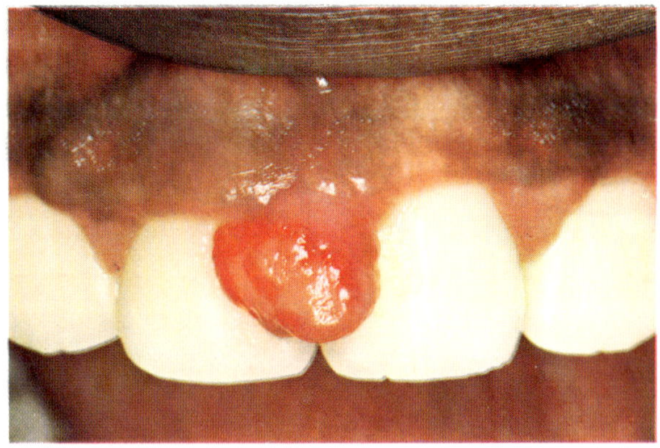

309 Ossifying fibrous epulis Excision biopsy and histological examination of the bright red lump attached to the interdental papilla between the maxillary central incisors in this 16 year old boy showed it to be an ossifying fibrous epulis. This lesion is a variant of a fibrous epulis which has a greater tendency to recur.

310

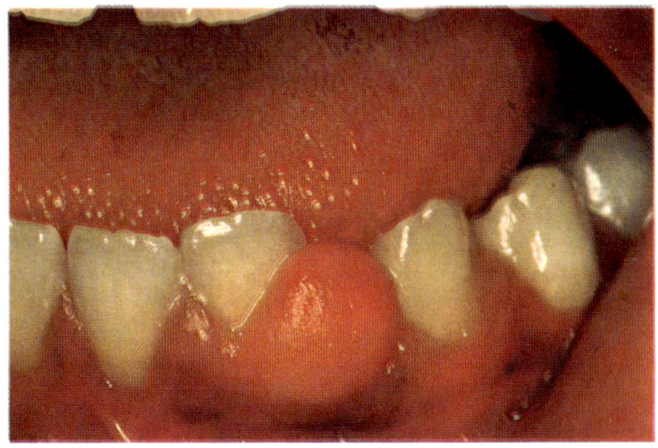

310 Ossifying fibrous epulis The localised swelling of the gingival margin and papilla between the left lateral incisor and canine had been present for some months in this 9 year old girl. A similar lesion had been excised from the same site several years earlier. Radiographs showed evidence of calcification within the swelling and excision biopsy confirmed the diagnosis of an ossifying fibrous epulis.

311

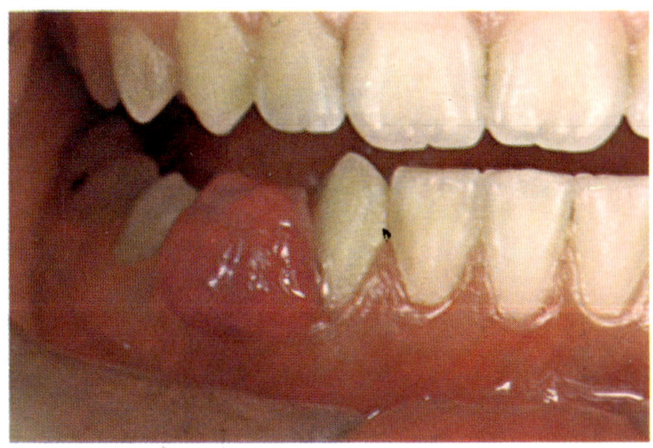

311 Pyogenic granuloma An adolescent presented with this pedunculated bright red swelling attached to the gingiva between the mandibular canine and first premolar. The lesion was excised and the area cauterised. The histological report was that of a pyogenic granuloma.

312

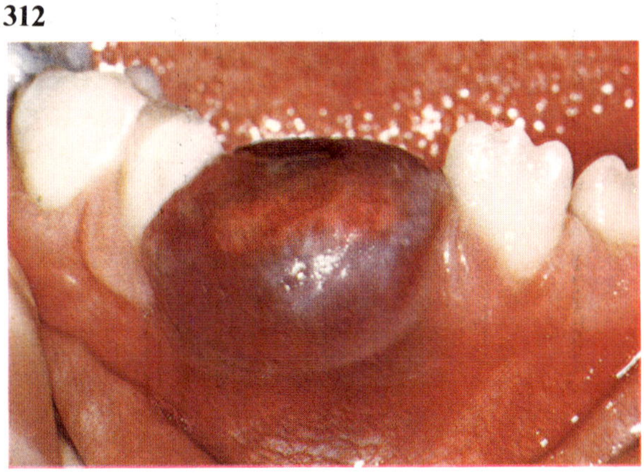

312 Giant cell epulis The maroon-coloured swelling on the gingiva in the mandibular right incisor region of this 7 year old boy had been present for 3 weeks and bled readily when touched. Excision biopsy confirmed the diagnosis of a giant cell epulis. A similar lesion had been removed from his 8 year old brother one year previously.

313 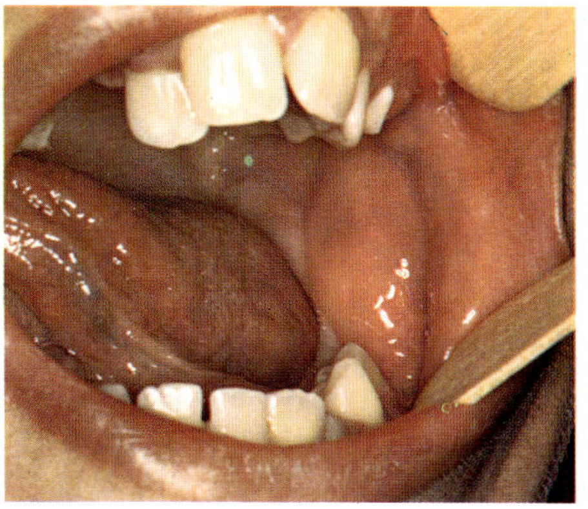

313 Plexiform neurofibromatosis Intraoral appearance of the neurofibroma seen in **61**. The tumour is seen to involve the gingival tissues overlying the unerupted mandibular molars on the left side of the jaw.

314 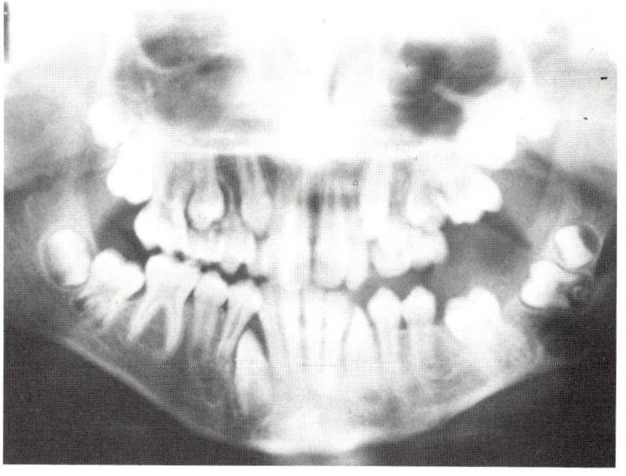

314 An orthopantomogram of the case seen in **313** shows the extent of bony involvement by the tumour with a large area of bony rarefaction in the left mandibular molar region and in the enlarged ascending ramus. These changes also involve the molar region of the maxilla on the same side.

b. Periodontal attachment

315 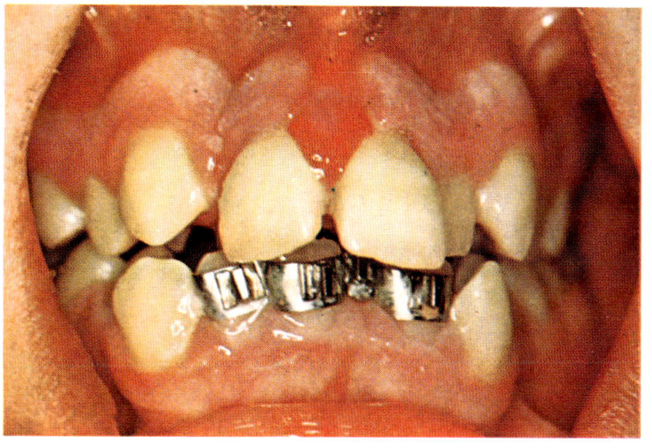

315 Periodontal trauma – elastic band injury Elastic bands are sometimes placed around maxillary central incisors to close a diastema, as in this teenager. The procedure is hazardous as the elastic bands may lead to gingival and periodontal tissue destruction through their apical migration.

316 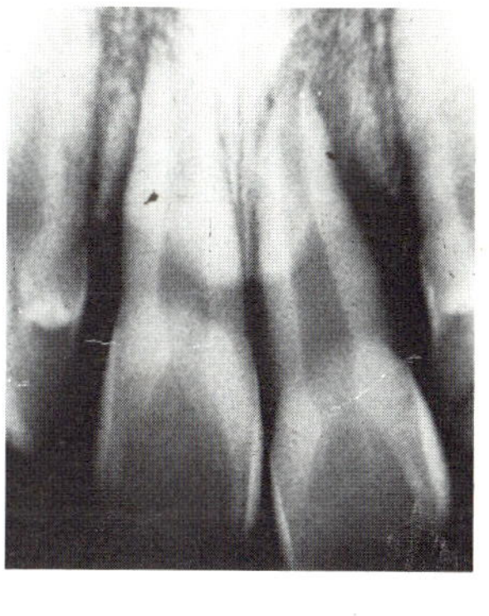

316 A radiograph of the case seen in **315** shows the extent of alveolar bony loss.

317

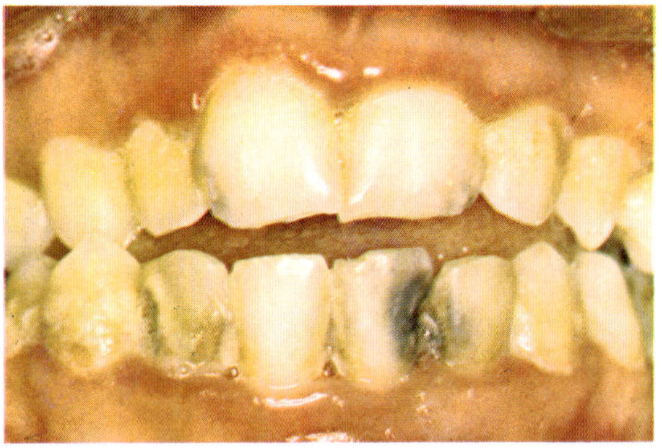

317 Down's syndrome (Mongolism, Trisomy 21) The neglected state of the dentition evident in a 14 year old severely subnormal girl with Down's syndrome is typical for many with this chromosomal anomaly. Both the plaque dependent diseases of caries and periodontitis are advanced in this patient.

318

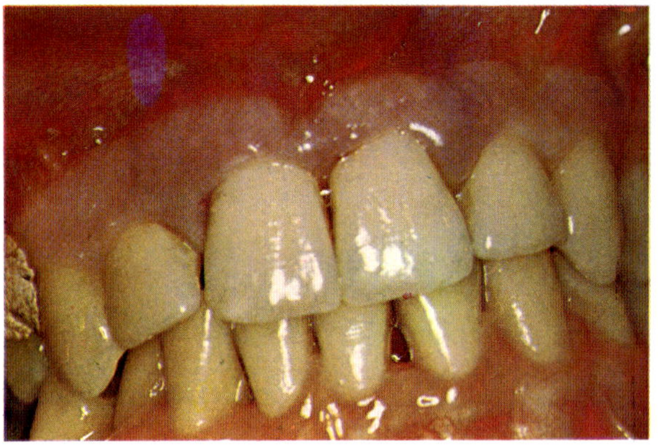

318 Juvenile periodontitis (Periodontosis) The clinical appearance of an adolescent with juvenile periodontitis may be misleading.

319

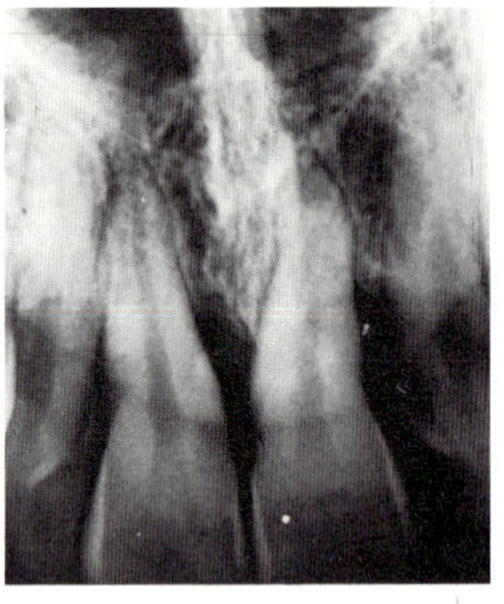

319 A radiograph from the patient seen in **318** shows the typical marked loss of alveolar bone around the maxillary incisor teeth.

320

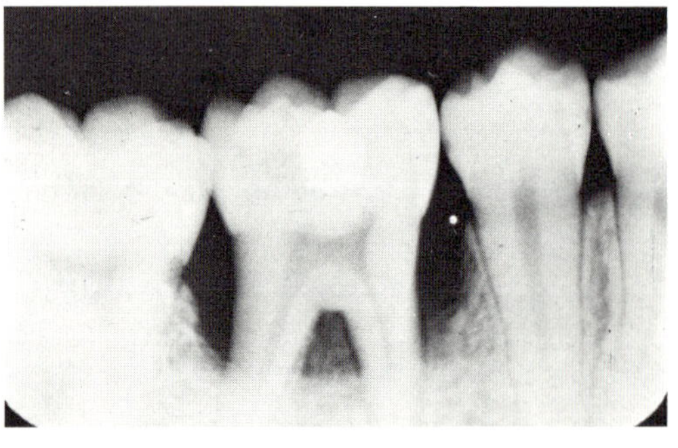

320 Juvenile periodontitis (Periodontosis) The gross destruction of alveolar bone around the first permanent molar is another characteristic feature of juvenile periodontitis.

321, 322 Juvenile periodontitis (Periodontosis) Radiographs showing the characteristic alveolar bony loss in the incisor and first molar regions in a 15 year old girl with this grossly destructive form of periodontal disease.

321

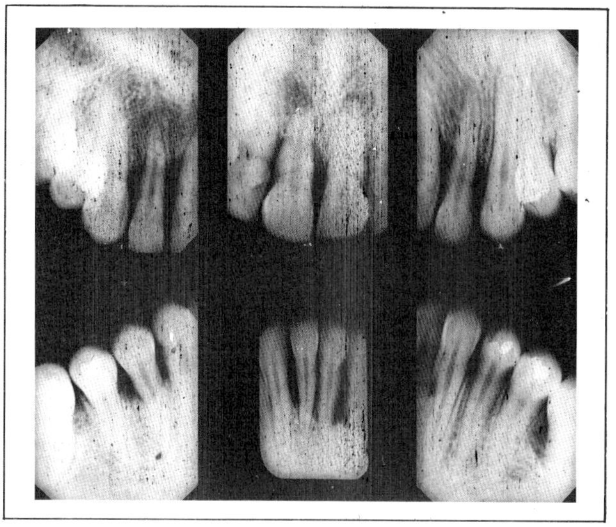

322

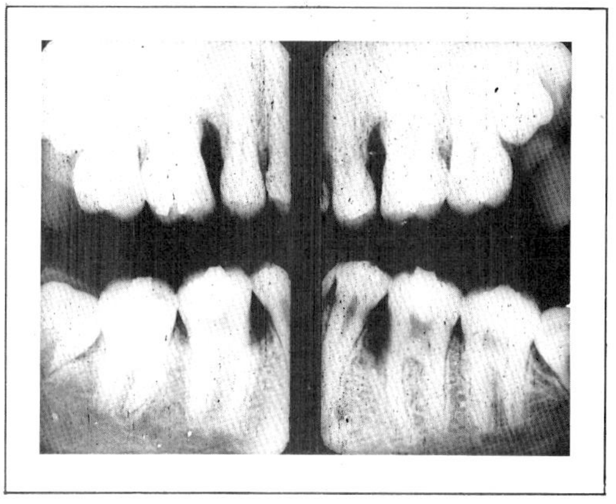

323 Juvenile periodontitis (Periodontosis) This 10 year old Pakistani girl with juvenile periodontitis shows a more generalised bony destruction around all her erupted permanent teeth.

323

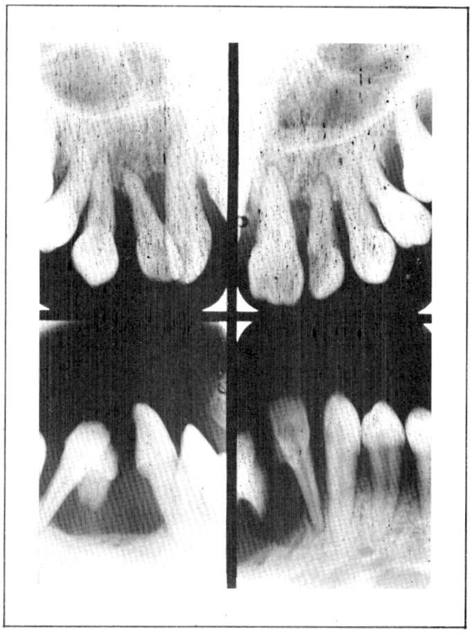

4. *The oral mucosa*

a. Lips

324

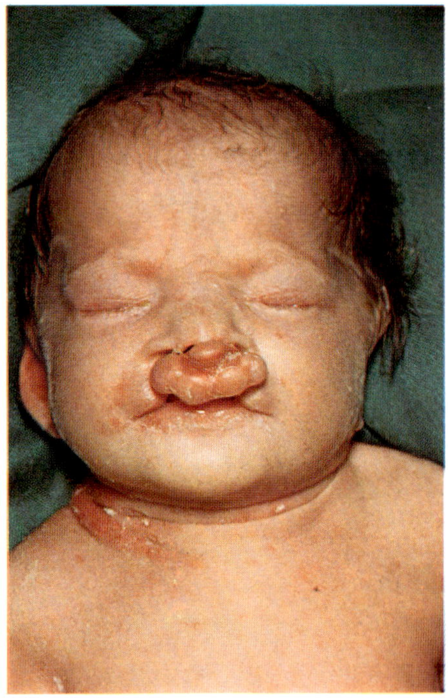

324 Cleft lip and palate Newly born baby with bilateral cleft lip and palate. Note the typical nasal deformity seen in this defect.

325

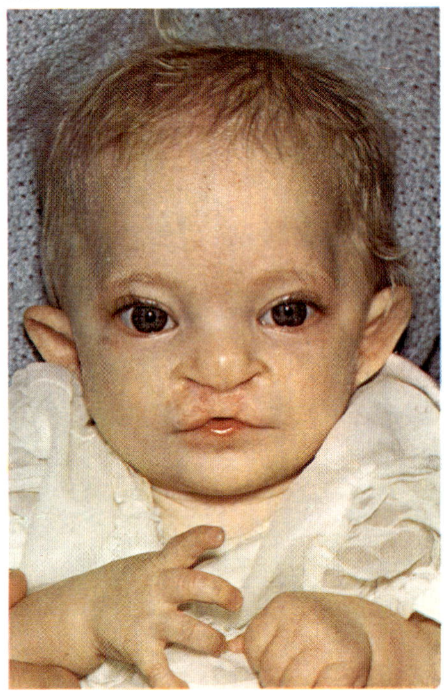

325 Cleft lip and palate Same child seen in **324** after successful repair of cleft lip.

326 **Verruca vulgaris (Infective papilloma, wart)** This 10 year old boy was already under treatment for plantar warts. The small papillomatous lesion on the mucosal surface of the upper lip had been present for 5 months.

326

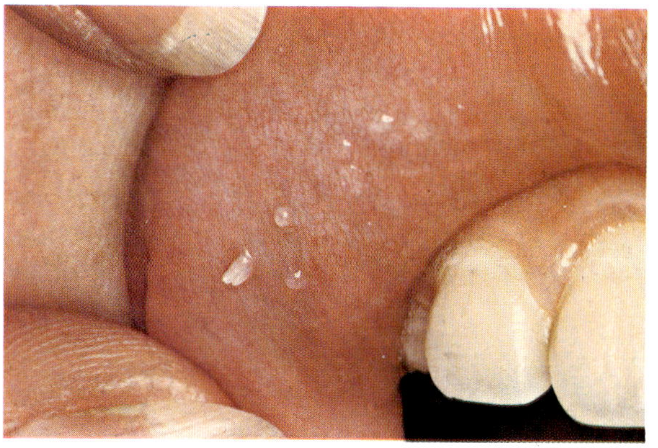

327 Excision biopsy of the lesion seen in **326** examined under E.M. shows the typical intra-nuclear virons. (×41,400)

327

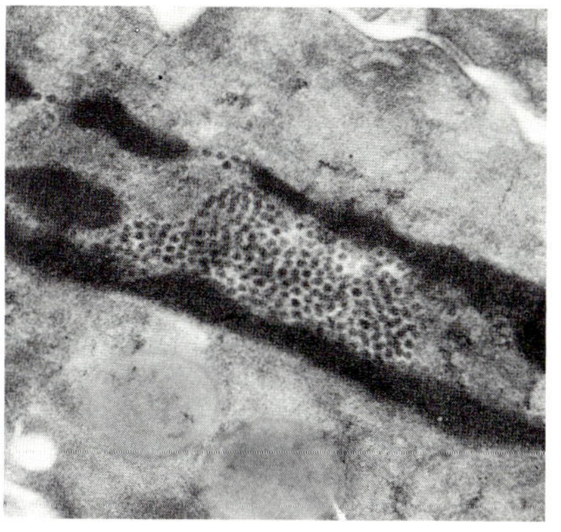

328 **Acute herpetic gingivostomatitis** In a 2 year old child multiple superficial ulcers on the mucosal surface of the lower lip each surrounded by a bright red halo, associated with an acute gingivitis, are indicative of a primary infection by the herpes simplex virus. (See **465**)

328

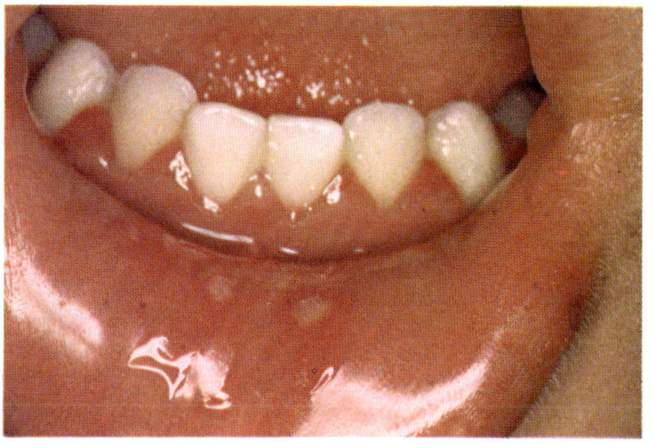

329 **Recurrent herpes labialis** The encrusted lesion at the muco-cutaneous border of the upper lip is characteristic of recurrent infection with herpes simplex virus. Note also the two warts affecting the lower lip.

329

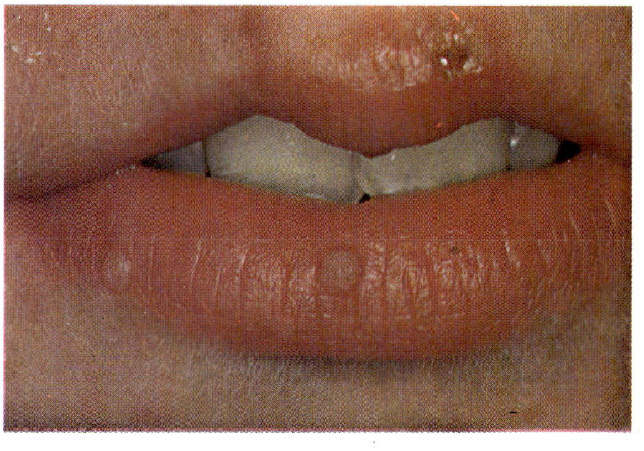

330 Recurrent herpetiform ulceration This 13 year old girl has suffered from recurrent oral ulceration for the past year with attacks every 2 months. The mucosal surface of the upper lip shows four small superficial herpetiform ulcers. There is no evidence to suggest these lesions are caused by the herpes simplex virus and the aetiology is unknown. These lesions respond rapidly to local treatment with tetracycline.

330

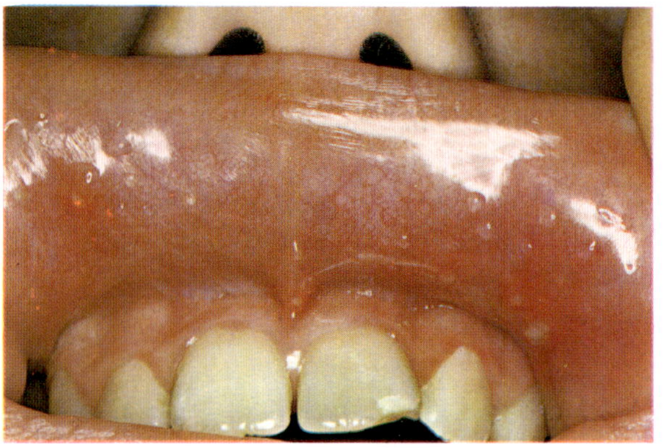

331, 332 Traumatic ulceration A lip sucking habit in which the lower lip was held behind the maxillary right lateral incisor was sufficiently traumatic to cause chronic ulceration of the mucosal surface in this teenage boy.

331

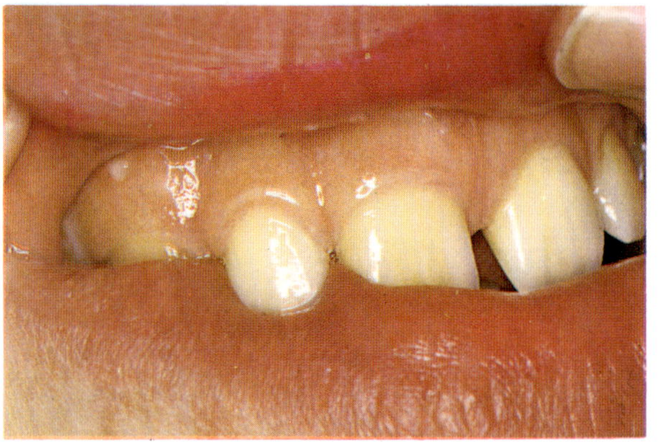

332

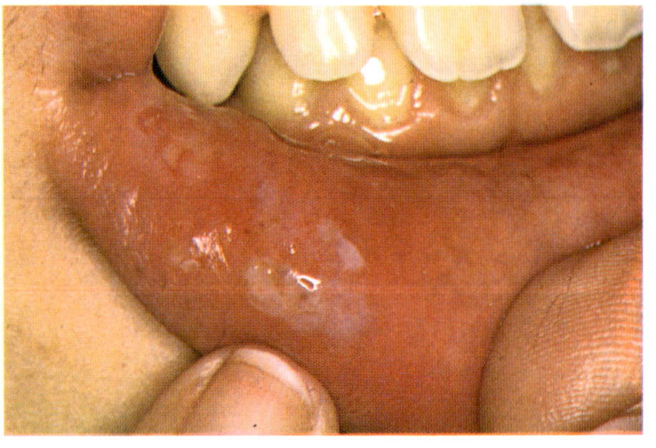

333 Laceration An intraoral laceration of the mucosa of the lower lip in this $2\frac{1}{2}$ year old child resulted in a full-thickness 'through and through' perforation of the lip.

333

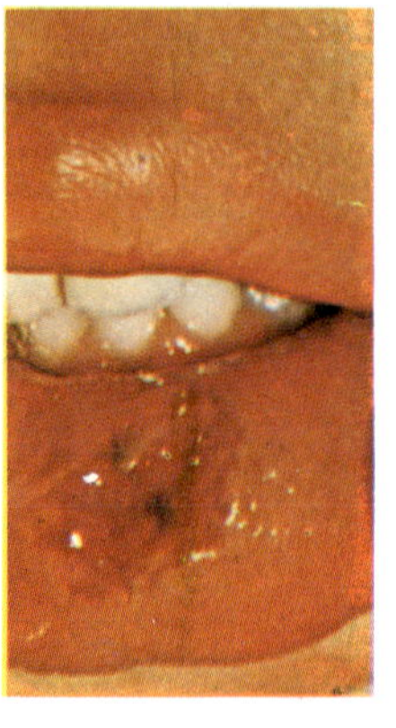

334

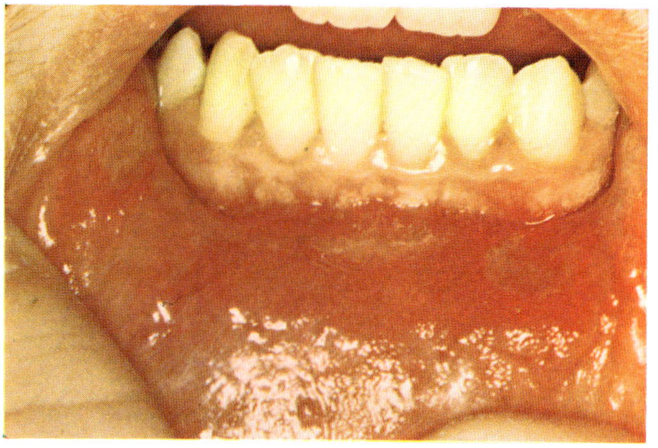

334 Recurrent aphthous ulceration Recurrent oral ulceration affecting the non-keratinised mucosal surfaces of the lips, cheeks and ventral surface of the tongue (see **419**) has been causing severe discomfort to this 13 year old girl for the past 3 years. The ulcers affecting the mucosal surface of the lower lip have been present for over 4 weeks. Fibrous scarring, from the healing of previous ulcers, is also present at the depth of the labial sulcus. This severe form of recurrent oral ulceration has been described as the major type to distinguish it from the simple form of minor aphthous ulceration.

335

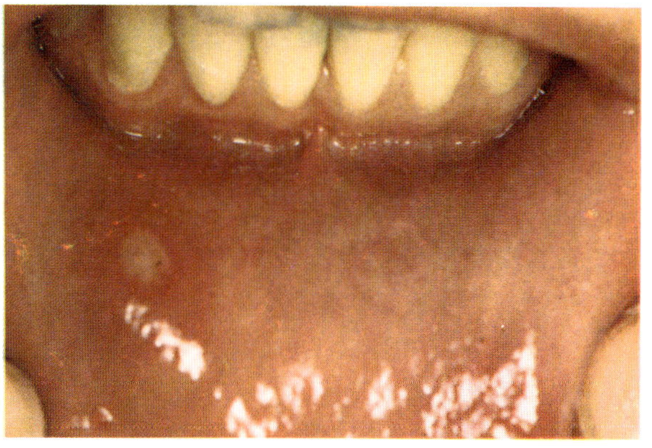

335 Aphthous ulcer (Canker sore) A typical simple or minor form of aphthous ulceration of the lower lip mucosa with a yellowish-white centre surrounded by an intensely red halo. These painful lesions usually heal in 5–7 days without scarring.

336

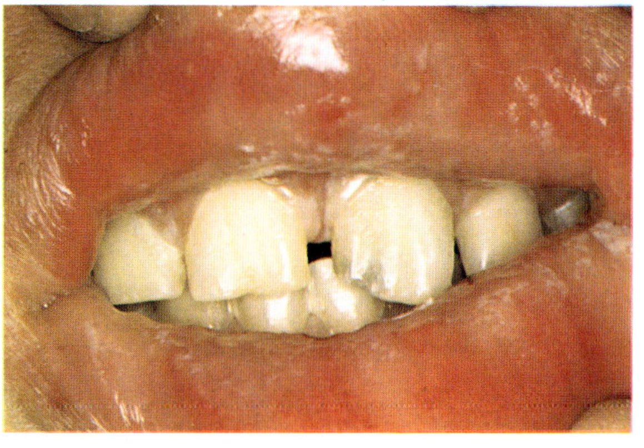

336 Acute candidiasis Two types of acute lesion produced by infection with Candida albicans are affecting the mucosal surfaces of the lips of this 12 year old boy. The bright red shiny areas are evidence of acute atrophic candidiasis, and the smaller whitish plaques are typical of the acute pseudo-membranous lesions of thrush.

337

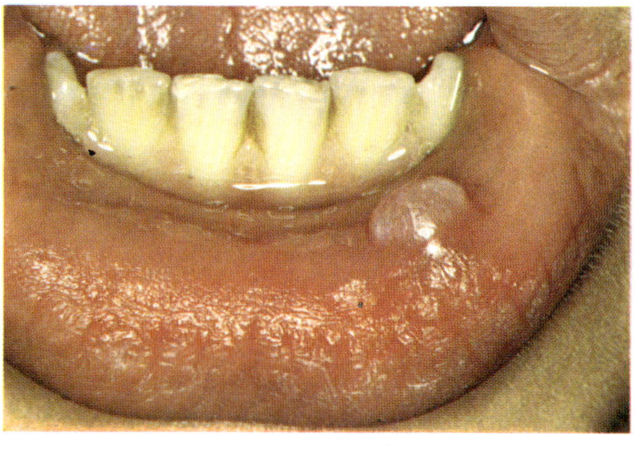

337 Mucocele The bluish translucent lesion on the mucosal surface of the lower lip is characteristic of a mucous extravasation or retention cyst (mucocele). A history of previous lip trauma is frequently obtained in such cases.

338 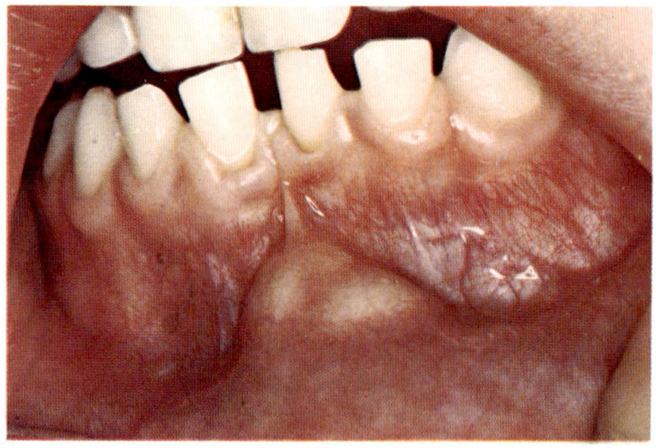

338 Dermoid cyst The swelling affecting the alveolar mucosa and the mucosal surface of the lower lip is a very rare example of a dermoid cyst in this location.

339 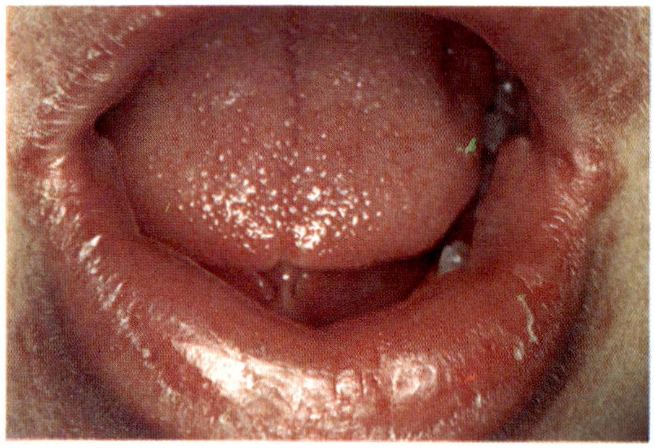

339 Crohn's disease (Cheilitis granulomatosa) The gross enlargement of the lower lip in this 8 year old girl has been present for about 6 months. The mucosal surface of the lip and cheek shows a 'cobblestone' appearance. Excision biopsy suggested the possible diagnosis of Crohn's disease, which was later confirmed by histological examination of an excised anal tag.

340 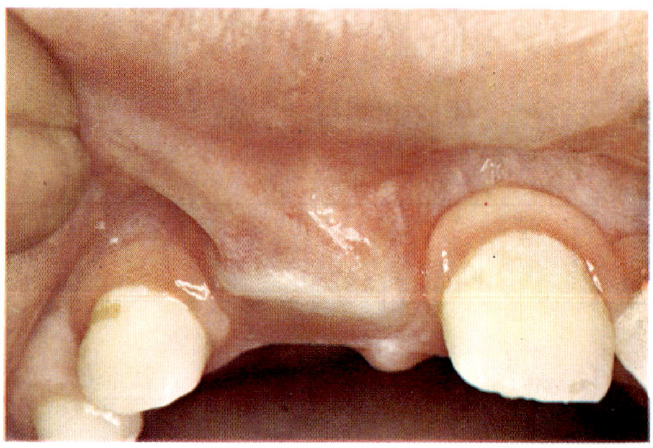

340 Ectopic eruption of central incisor Ectopic eruption of a maxillary right central incisor into the upper lip is made obvious by stretching of the mucosal surface.

b. Alveolar mucosa

341 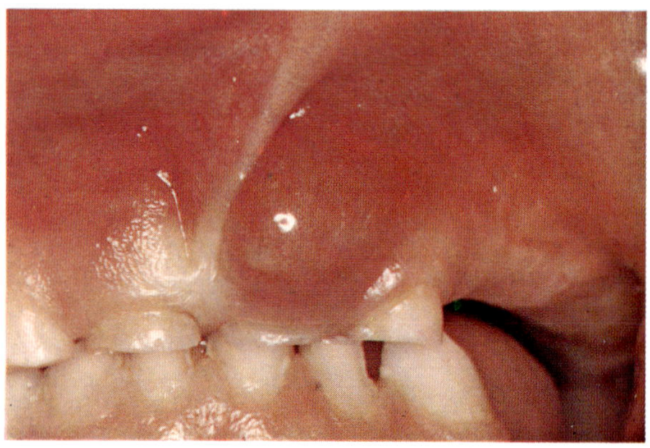

341 Dentoalveolar abscess A subacute dentoalveolar abscess is present in the labial sulcus overlying the left primary central incisor. All the maxillary incisors are severely worn by attrition and the pulp of the left central incisor has become exposed by this process.

342

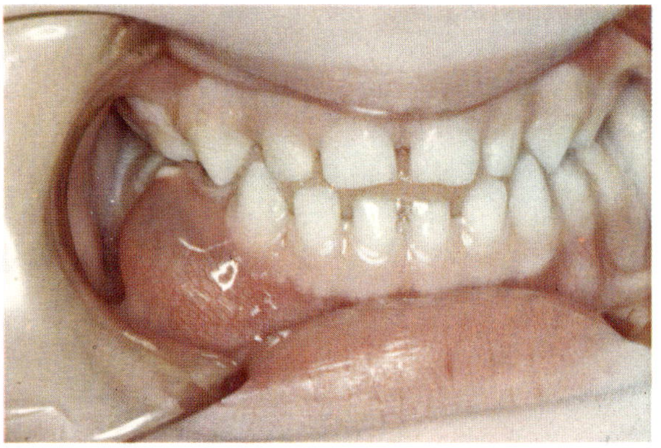

342 Radicular cyst The large bluish-red swelling in the buccal sulcus is a radicular cyst associated with a cariously exposed and non-vital first primary molar.

343

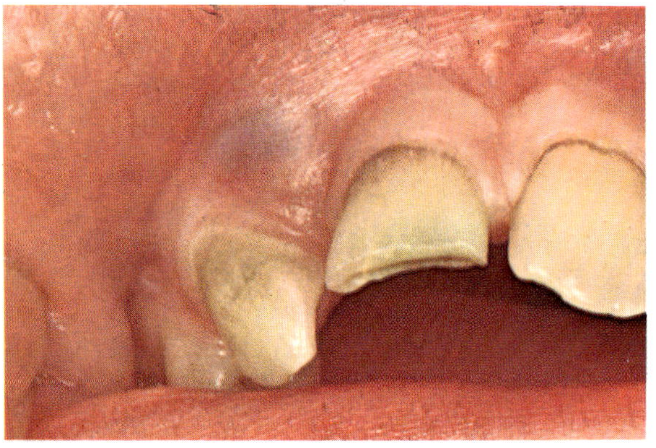

343 Residual radicular cyst The bluish lesion of the alveolar mucosa in the right lateral incisor region of the maxilla is evidence of a residual radicular cyst. Previous trauma was responsible for coronal fractures of the permanent right central and lateral incisors. The lateral incisor had become non-vital and was extracted, leaving a radicular cyst in situ.

344

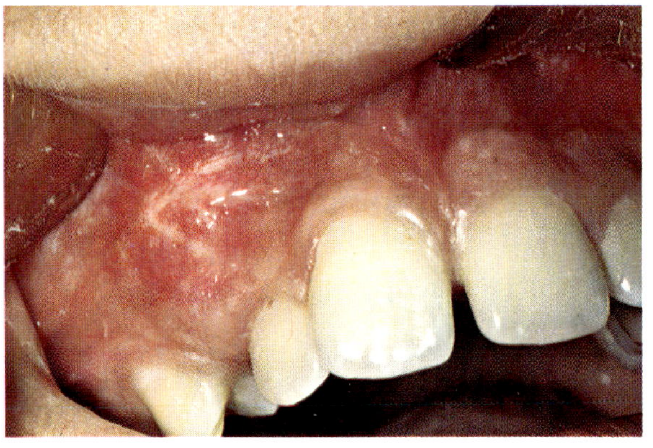

344 Post surgical scar The posteriorly directed V-shaped fibrous tissue scar of the alveolar mucosa overlying the maxillary right lateral incisor is a permanent record of earlier surgery for the removal of a radicular cyst.

345

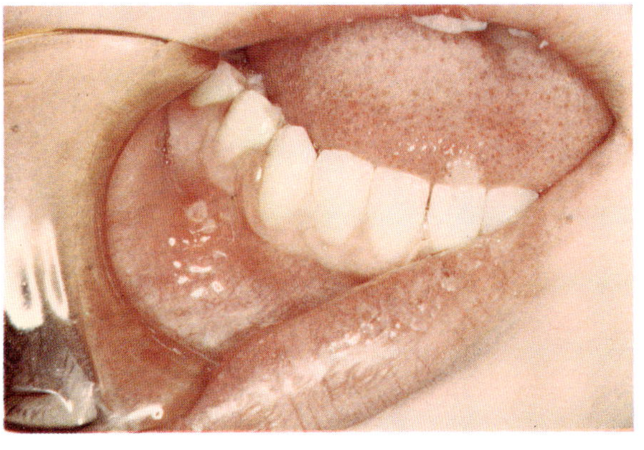

345 Acute herpetic gingivostomatitis Herpetic ulcer of the alveolar mucosa in a relatively mild primary attack of herpes simplex virus infection.

346

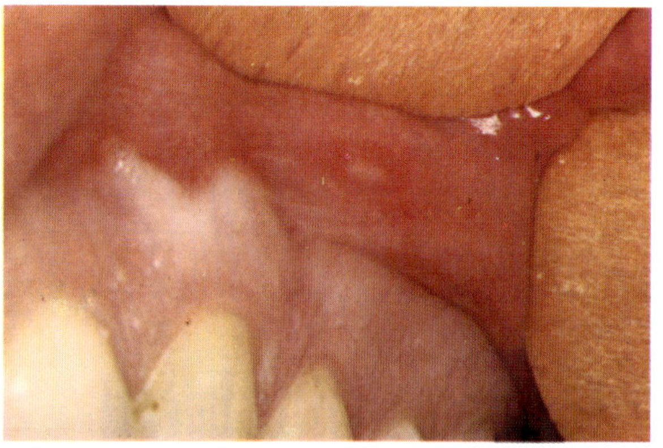

346 Hand, foot and mouth disease This small superficial ulcer of the alveolar mucosa is only one aspect of a more generalised infection by the Coxsackie virus affecting the oral mucosa and the skin of the hands and feet. (See **467** and **475**)

347

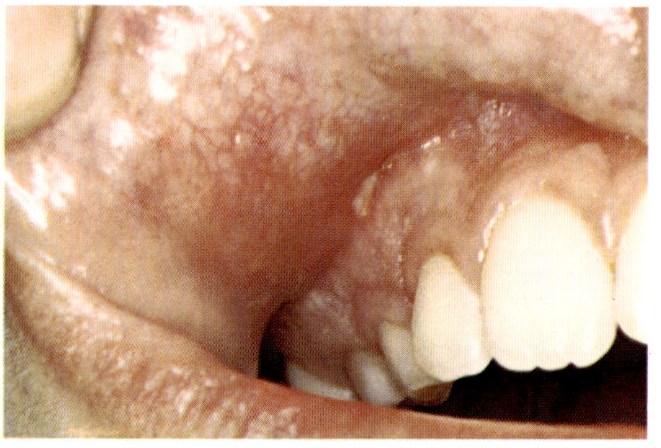

347 Aphthous ulcer Aphthous ulceration of the alveolar mucosa is seen in this 9 year old boy at the depth of the upper buccal sulcus. There appeared to be an association between the ulcers and the ingestion of fruit, as each time he consumed tomatoes or oranges he developed an ulcer shortly afterwards.

c. Cheeks

348

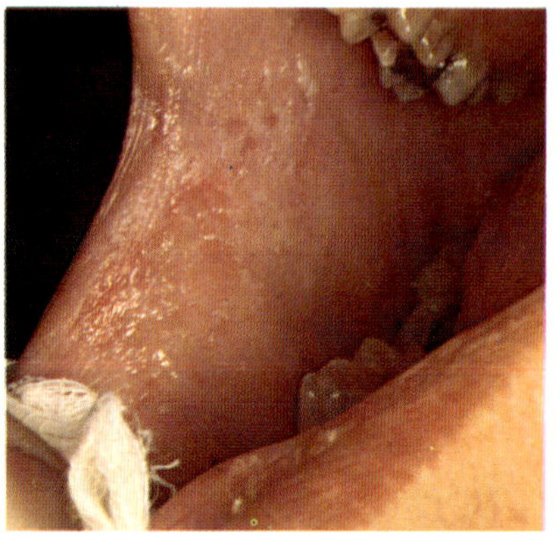

348 White sponge naevus The buccal mucosa of the cheek in this 13 year old girl has a whitish pebbled appearance which is known as a white sponge naevus, a developmental anomaly of the oral mucosa which remains benign throughout life.

349

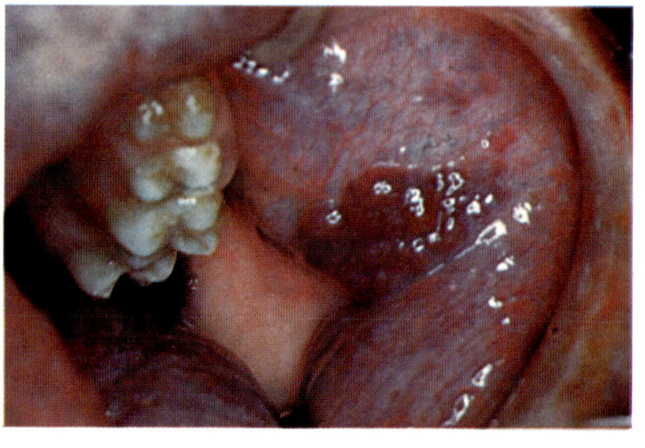

349 Encephalofacial angiomatosis (Sturge-Weber syndrome) The oral manifestations of encephalofacial angiomatosis (Sturge-Weber syndrome) are well illustrated in this child with gross distortion of the left cheek by haemangiomatous malformations.

350 Lym hangioma The entire buccal mucosa of the right cheek in this boy shows the typical pebbled appearance of a lymphangioma. The fluid-filled spaces of the swelling transilluminate brilliantly. (See **37**)

350

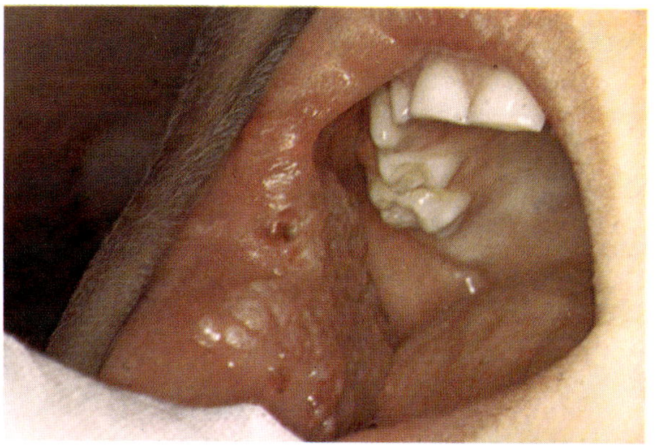

351 Lichen planus The characteristic whitish reticular lesions of lichen planus are affecting the mucosa of the right cheek in this teenager.

351

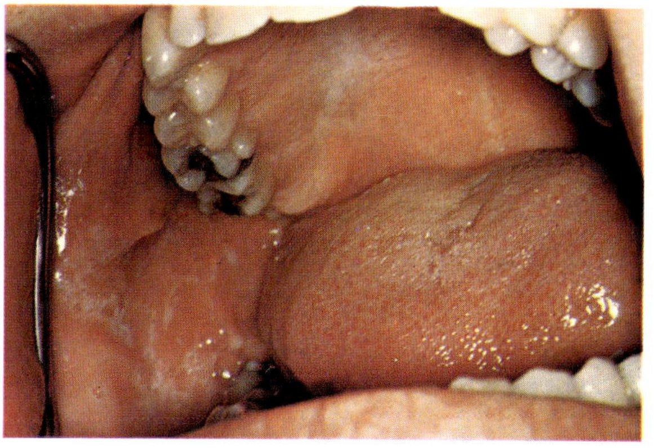

352 Aspirin burn The whitish necrotic mucosa and fibrous scarring of the cheek in this adolescent are the result of considerable irritation from the holding of aspirin tablets in the buccal sulcus.

352

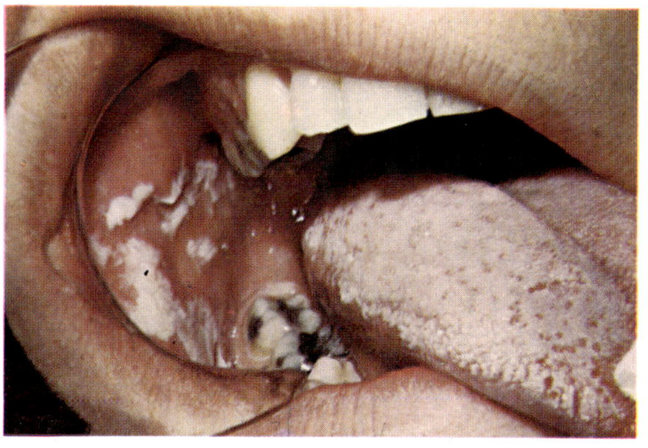

353 Cheek biting While the biting of lips and tongue is the most frequent sequela to the administration of local analgesics in the lower jaw, traumatised cheeks are not uncommon. This child shows the typical appearance of healing following the biting of an anaesthetised cheek.

353

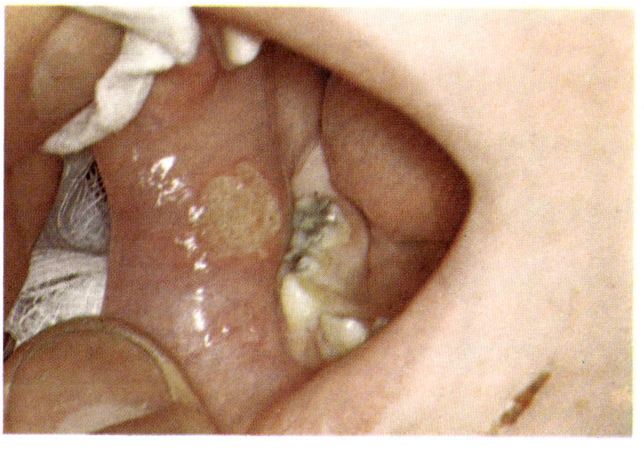

354

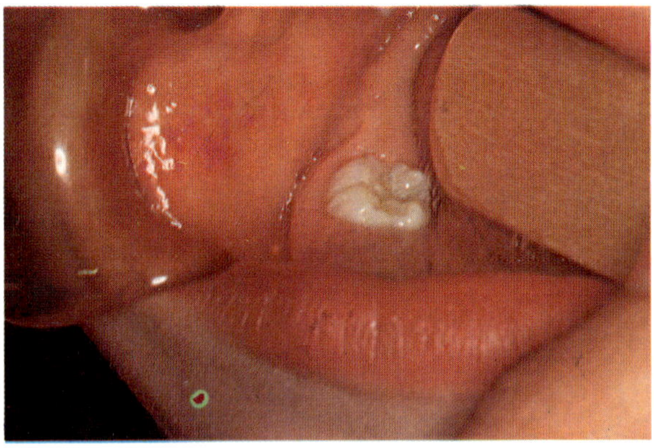

354 Cheek biting The small ulcers of the cheek mucosa in this child lie parallel to the line of the occlusion and are caused by habitual cheek biting. Emotional instability and occlusal disharmony are two factors which may predispose to such self-inflicted trauma.

355

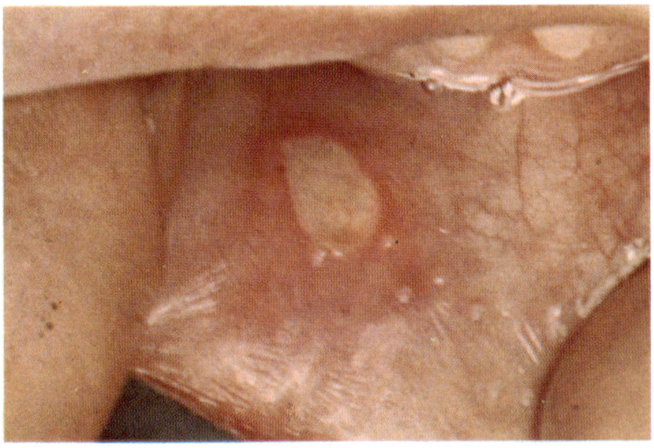

355 Aphthous ulcer The superficial lesion of the cheek mucosa immediately inside the commissure of the lips is typical for the minor form of aphthous ulceration. It is affecting the non-keratinised mucosa, has a yellowish-white base with surrounding area of erythema and is in a site frequently affected by such lesions. Ulcers of this type usually heal within a week without evidence of scarring.

356

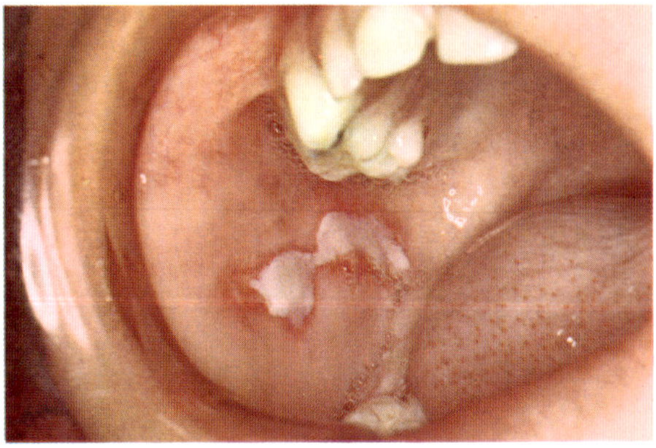

356 Staphylococcal ulceration The unusual ulceration of the right cheek in this young child proved on bacterial culture to be associated with coagulase positive Staphylococcus aureus infection. It is a superficial form of mucosal ulceration with an irregular margin, yellow slough and a fine line of surrounding erythema. It responded rapidly to antibiotic therapy.

357

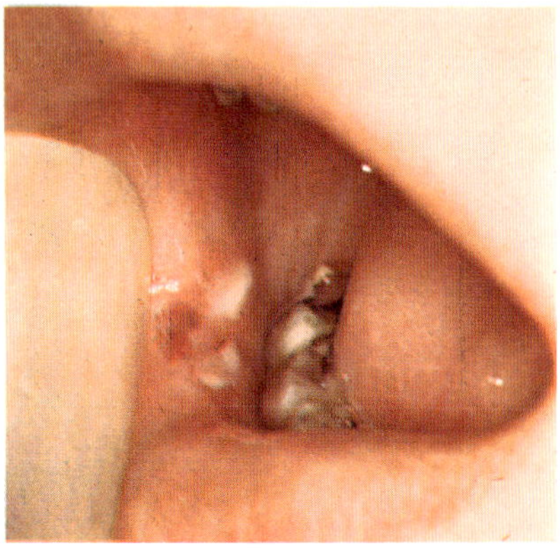

357 Epidermolysis bullosa dystrophica The ulceration and whitish sloughing of the cheek mucosa in this child are associated with bullous lesions of the skin especially on the upper and lower limbs. Oral lesions of this type are most frequently seen in the autosomal recessive variety of epidermolysis bullosa dystrophica. (See **464**)

d. Floor of mouth

358

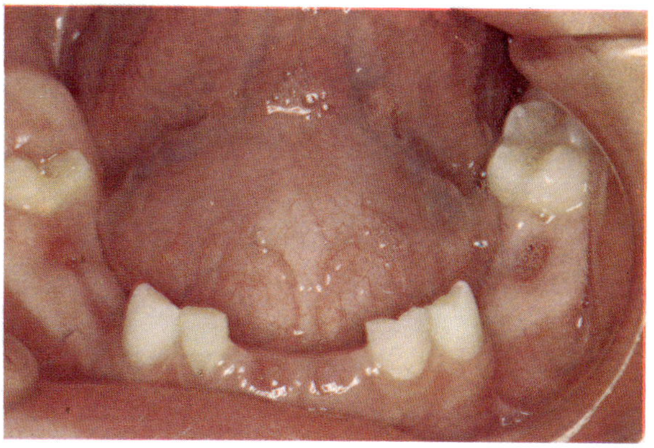

358 Sublingual dermoid cyst A 6 year old boy presented with this large midline swelling in the floor of the mouth and was having difficulty in protruding his tongue. The swelling was the same colour as the remainder of the mucosa, non-tender and non-transilluminable. Excision biopsy confirmed the diagnosis of a dermoid cyst.

359

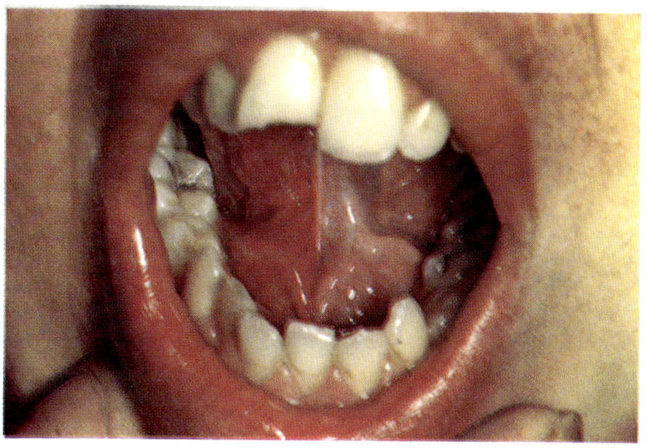

359 Capillary haemangioma This capillary haemangioma is involving the mucosa in the floor of the mouth unilaterally. The facial skin on the same side is affected by a 'port-wine stain' or naevus flammeus.

360

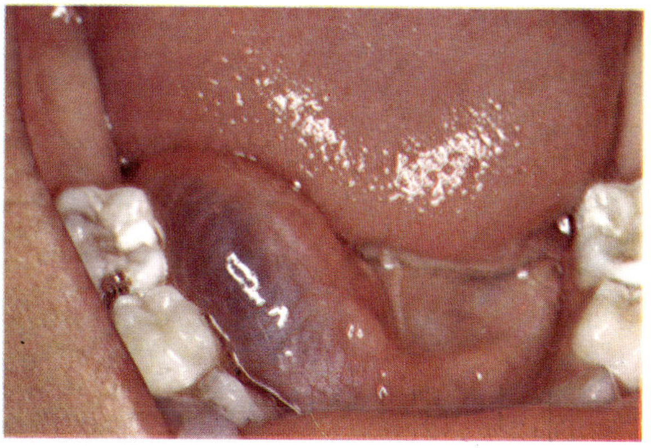

360 Mucocele (Ranula) The unilateral bluish translucent lesion in this 4 year old girl was of recent onset and non-tender. It transilluminated brilliantly. Marsupialisation into the floor of the mouth was undertaken and the biopsy report confirmed the diagnosis of a mucous extravasation cyst. Mucoceles in this situation are given the descriptive title of ranula.

361

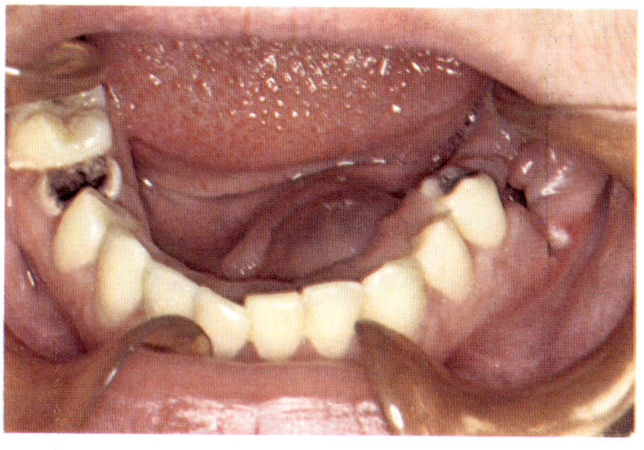

361 Sublingual abscess This acutely tender and fluctuant sublingual abscess appears to have been initiated by the spread of infection from the socket of a recently extracted mandibular first permanent molar on the same side.

362

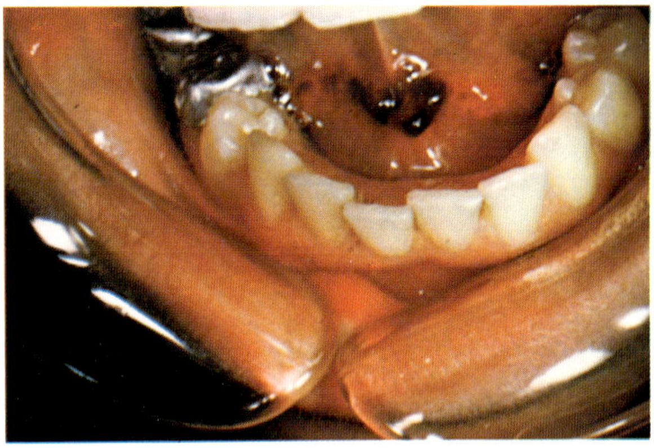

362 Haematoma A small haematoma in the floor of the mouth caused by trauma from a saliva ejector.

363

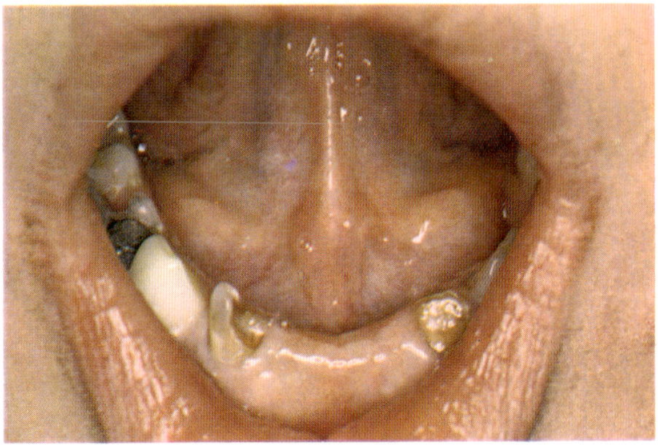

363 Congenital absence of submandibular salivary glands The unusual destruction of the mandibular primary incisors by rampant caries in this 4 year old boy drew attention to the congenital absence of the submandibular (Wharton's) duct orifices in the floor of the mouth, and the associated bilateral congenital absence of submandibular salivary glands.

364

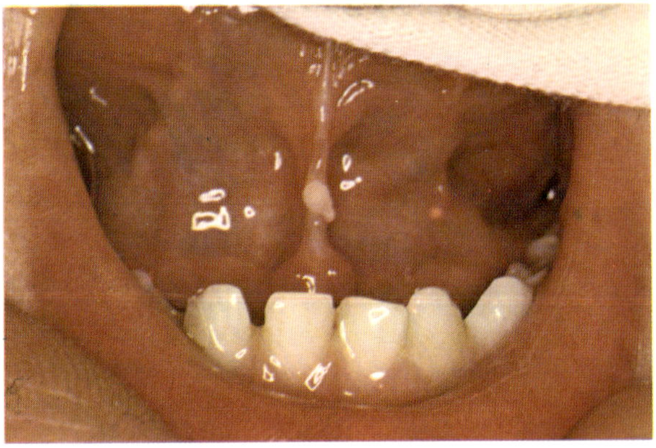

364 Ankyloglossia (Tongue tie) The marked sublingual frenum in this young child is associated with a limited protrusive ability of the tip of the tongue. In attempting to make protrusive movements the frenum has been ulcerated by the lower incisors.

365

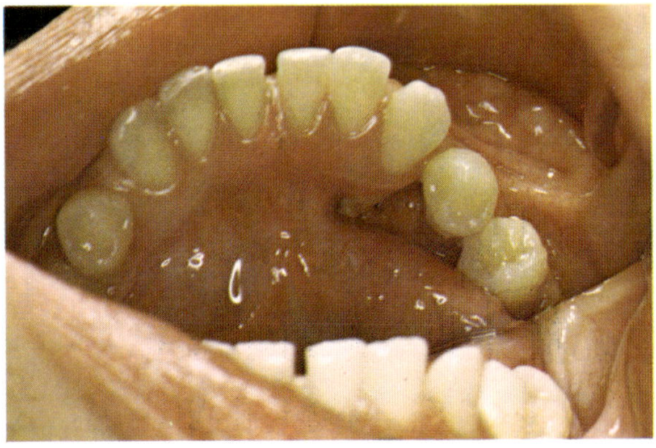

365 Histiocytosis X (Hand-Schüller-Christian type) The lingual aspect of the roots of the mandibular right canine and first premolar are exposed by necrosis of the overlying mucosa and bone in this teenage boy with Hand-Schüller-Christian disease. Other bony lesions were noted in the jaws, skull and femur, and he was suffering from diabetes insipidus. (See **439** and **440**)

366

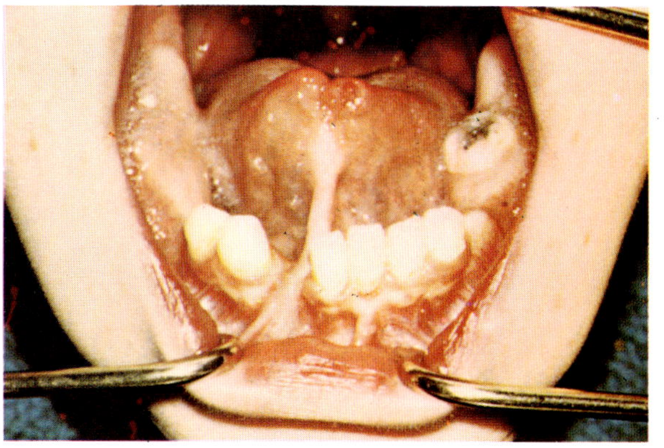

366 Orodigitofacial dysostosis (OFD syndrome) Clefting of the mandibular alveolus in the region of the missing right lateral incisor by a thick fibrous band extending from the lip to the tongue is the most prominent oral feature in this child with OFD syndrome. A lobulated tongue and tethering of the lip to the gingiva by further frena are two other features to be seen. (See **410** and **411**)

367

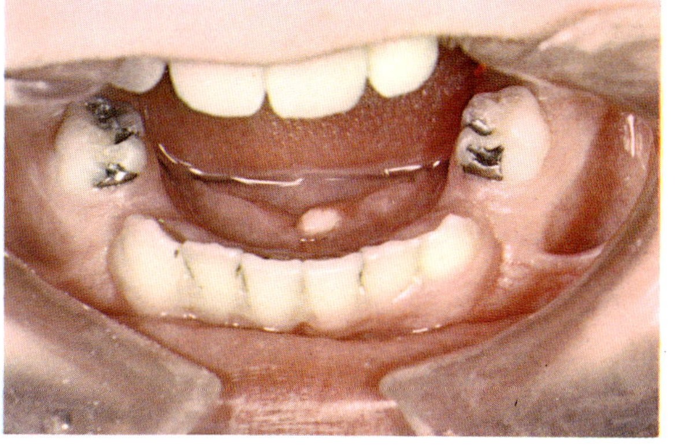

367 Submandibular calculus The whitish mass in the floor of the mouth of this 10 year old boy is due to the impaction of a calculus at the orifice of the left submandibular (Wharton's) duct.

368

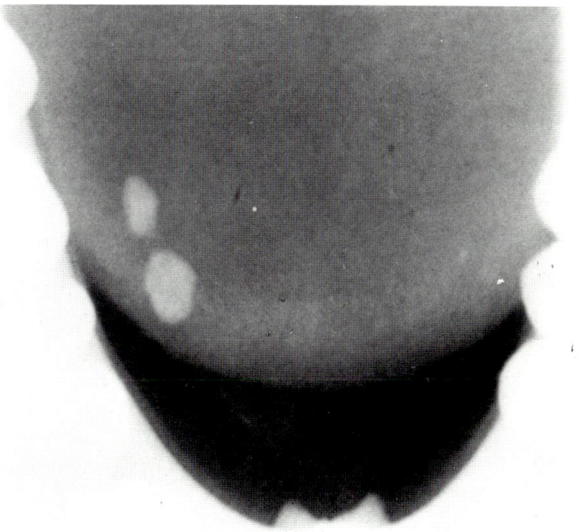

368 Submandibular calculus The occlusal radiograph illustrates the presence of a radiopaque calculus in the right submandibular (Wharton's) duct.

5. *The palate*

369 Unilateral cleft lip and palate A complete unilateral cleft of lip, alveolar process and palate.

369

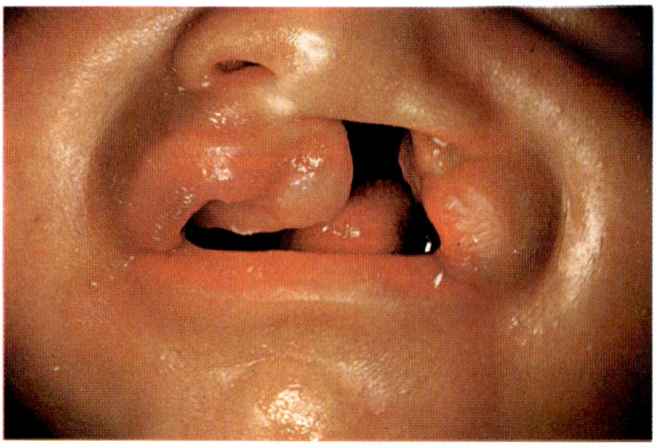

370 Bilateral cleft lip and palate A complete bilateral cleft of lip, alveolar process and palate.

370

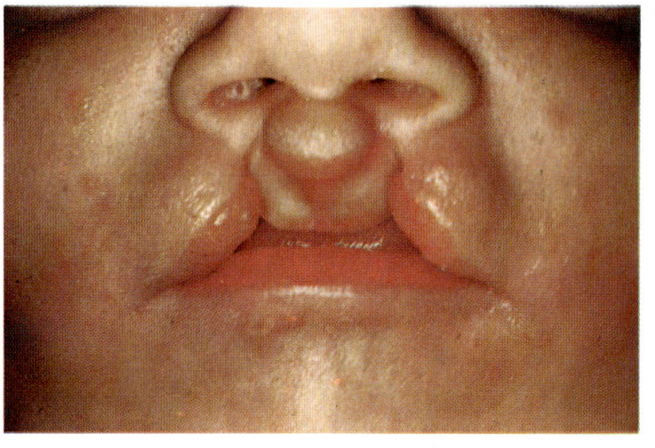

371 Partial cleft of soft and hard palate This child has an incomplete cleft of soft and hard palate.

371

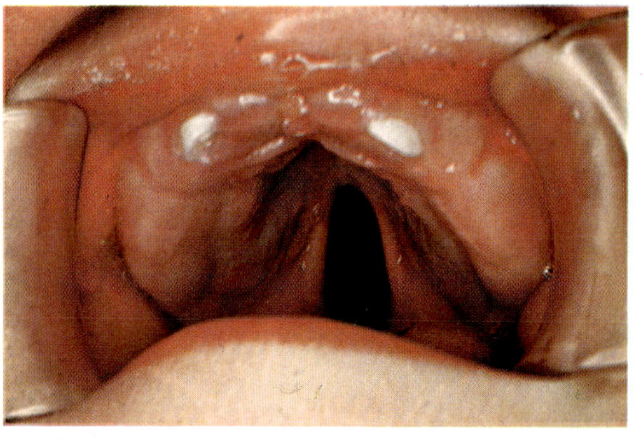

372

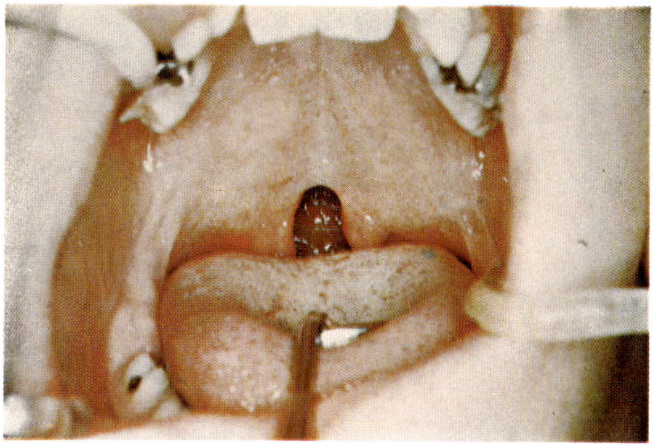

372 Isolated cleft of soft palate An isolated cleft of soft palate and uvula in a teenager.

373

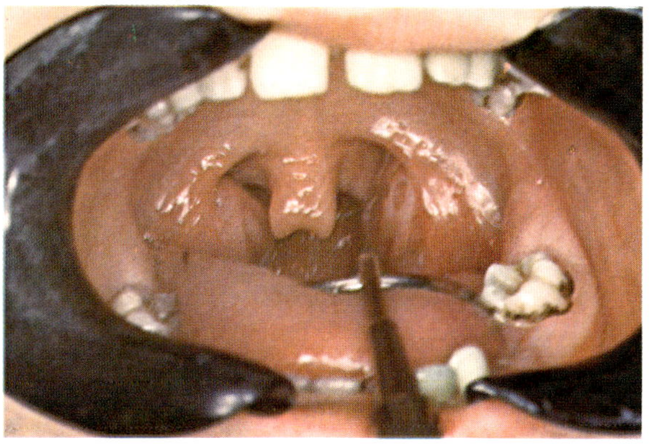

373 Bifid uvula This uvula has an abnormal cleavage.

374

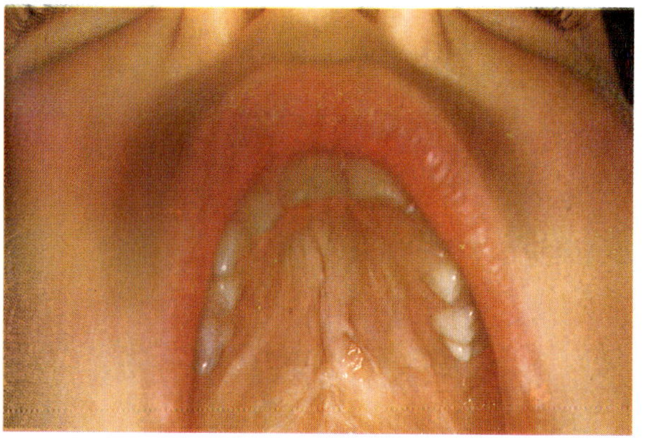

374 Repaired cleft palate Scar tissue resulting from the surgical repair of the cleft of hard and soft palates.

375

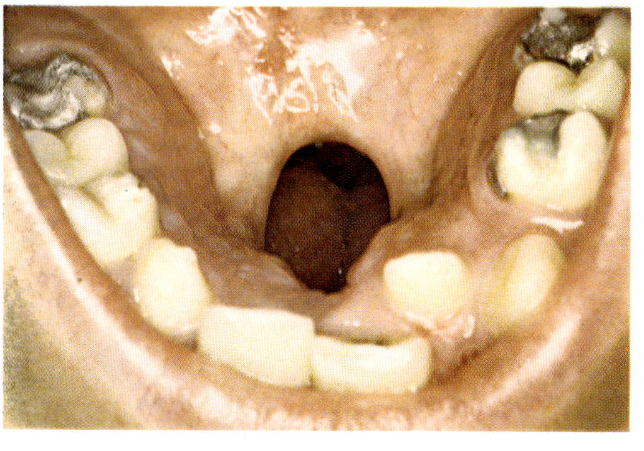

375 Incomplete repair of cleft palate This 14 year old boy has a residual defect in the hard palate after an incomplete repair of the soft and hard palates at the age of 2½ years.

376

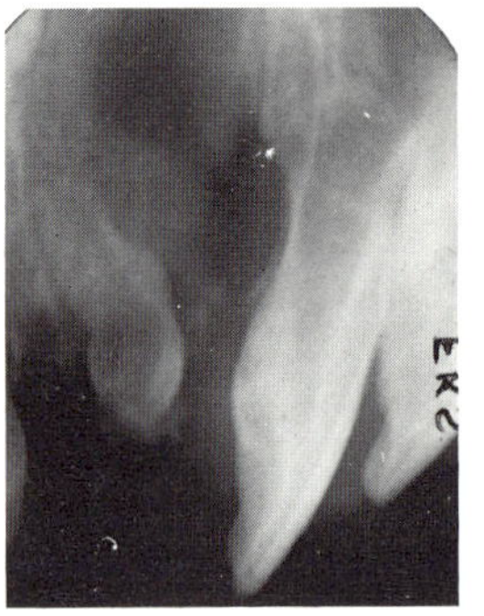

376 Alveolar cleft and dental anomaly An unerupted tooth with a conical crown and a dilacerated root is evident in the line of the alveolar cleft in this radiograph.

377

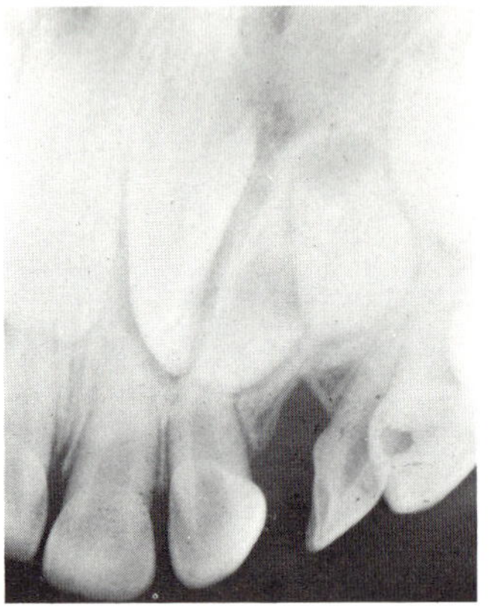

377 Partial alveolar cleft and dental anomaly This 5 year old boy with a repaired unilateral cleft lip presented with a supernumerary primary tooth erupting distal to a partial cleft of the alveolus. The radiograph shows the presence of an unerupted conical supernumerary tooth lying between the rotated permanent left central and lateral incisors.

378

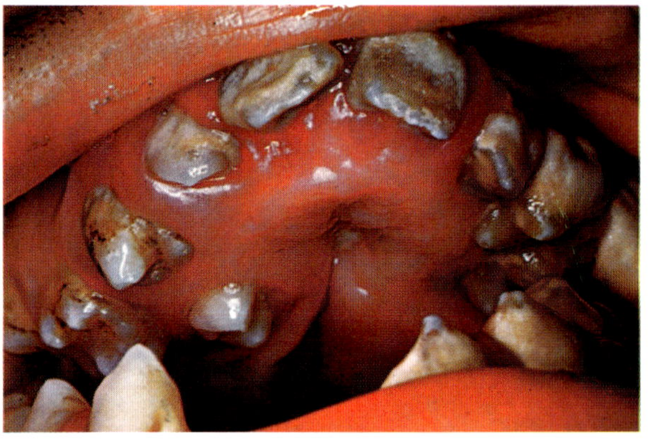

378 Acrocephalosyndactyly (Apert's syndrome) The abnormal palate in this patient with Apert's syndrome shows a distinct median furrow, marked thickening of the alveolar process, considerable crowding of the teeth and the ectopic eruption of the right second premolar. (See **7** and **476**)

379

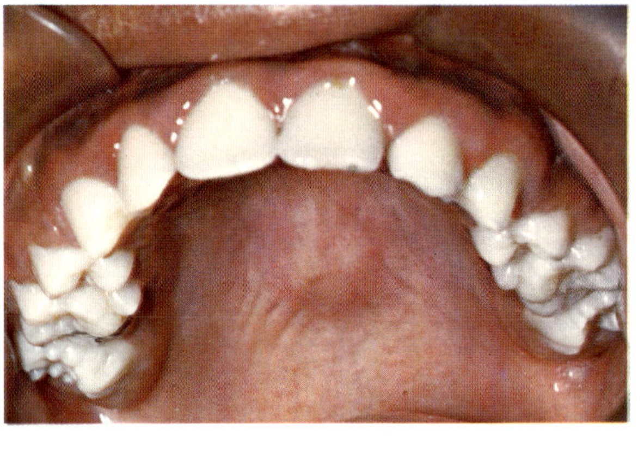

379 Torus palatinus An adolescent patient with a marked midline torus palatinus.

380 Marfan's syndrome The very high arched palate in this 3 year old girl with Marfan's syndrome is indented by the nasal septum. Long tapering fingers typical of arachnodactyly and considerable laxity of the temporomandibular joints were also noted. (See **459**)

380

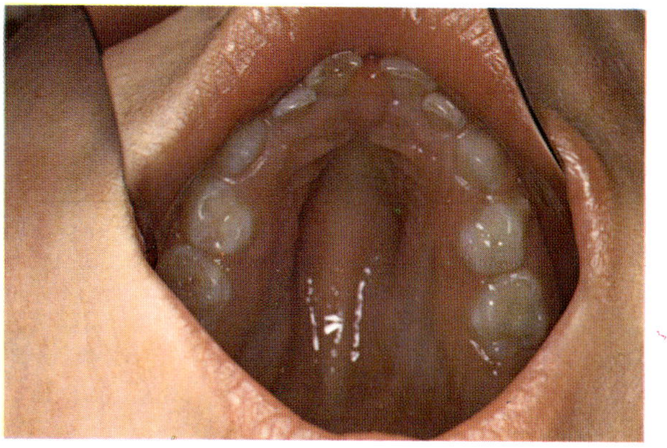

381 Palatal pit This 4 year old girl shows an unusual small midline defect in the mucosa of the hard palate immediately posterior to the incisive papilla.

381

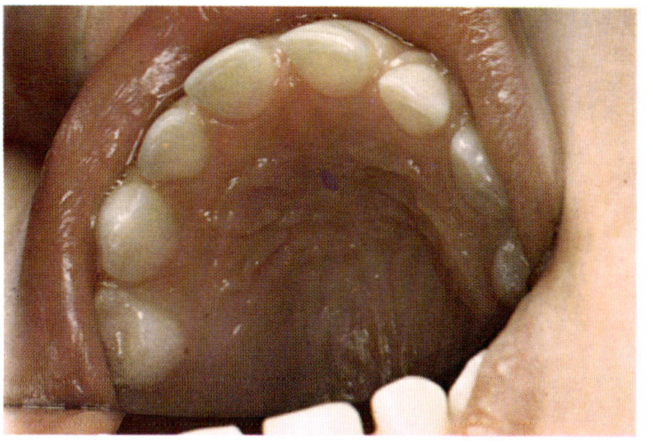

382 Electrical burn of palate The scarring and contraction of the hard palate in this 10 year old boy were caused by biting through a live electrical cord 7 years earlier and sustaining a severe burn. (See **412**)

382

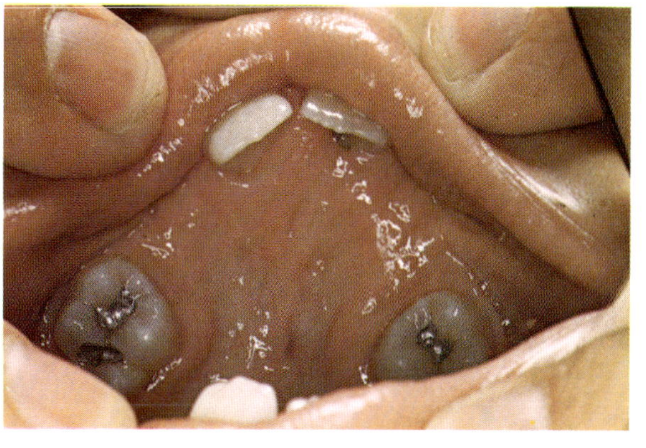

383 Junctional naevus The small pigmented lesion in the palatal mucosa adjacent to the left primary canine had been present for 17 months and recently increased in size. Excision biopsy showed the lesion to be a junctional naevus. These naevi may occasionally become malignant.

383

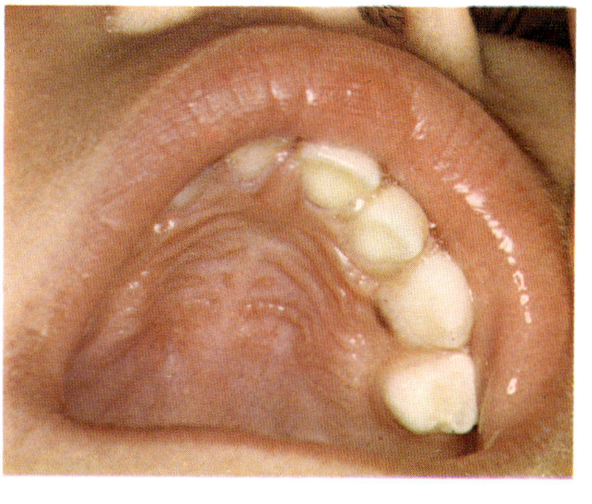

384 Cavernous haemangioma The bluish-red swelling involving the left side of the soft palate and cheek in this 15 year old boy is the visible evidence of a large cavernous haemangioma which extended upwards into the pterygoid space and backwards beneath the base of the skull. Attempts to ligate the afferent vessels of supply had failed. (See **27**)

384

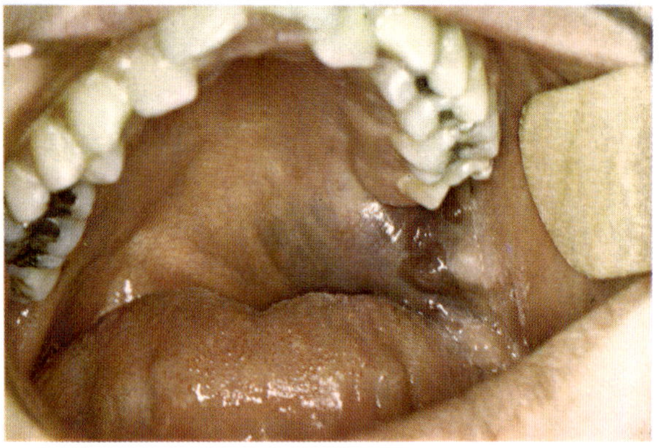

385 Mucous cyst of the palate Large mucous retention cyst of the palate in a newly born baby.

385

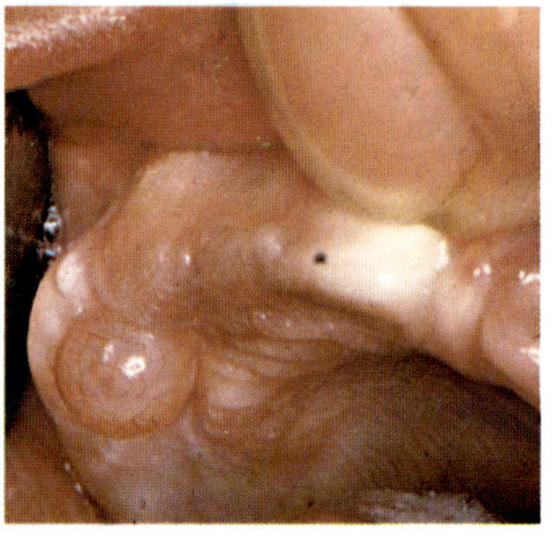

386 Palatal abscess Yellow pus may be seen beneath the palatal mucosa in this pointing abscess which is derived from a grossly carious, non-vital and infected first permanent molar.

386

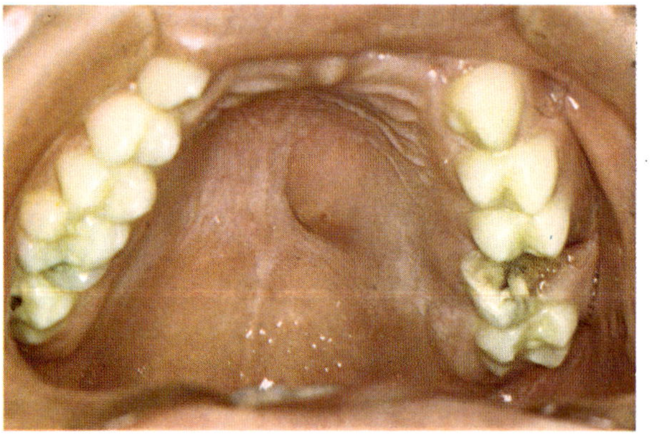

387 Acute herpetic gingivostomatitis The bright redness and swelling of the palatal gingiva in this patient is seen in association with acute herpetic gingivostomatitis.

387

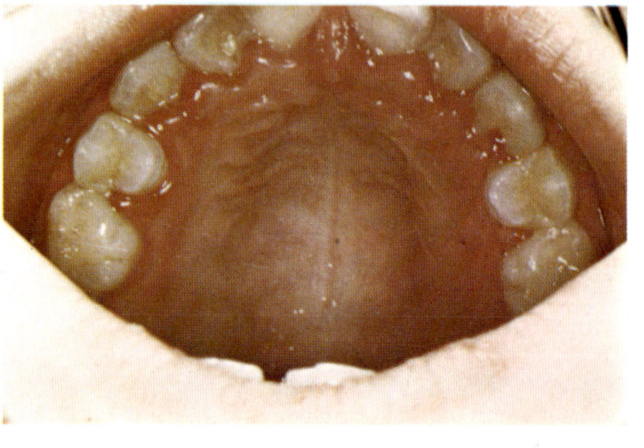

388 Acute herpetic gingivostomatitis The acute primary infection by the herpes simplex virus is limited in this patient to the mucosa on the left side of the hard palate where a collection of small ulcerative lesions is present.

388

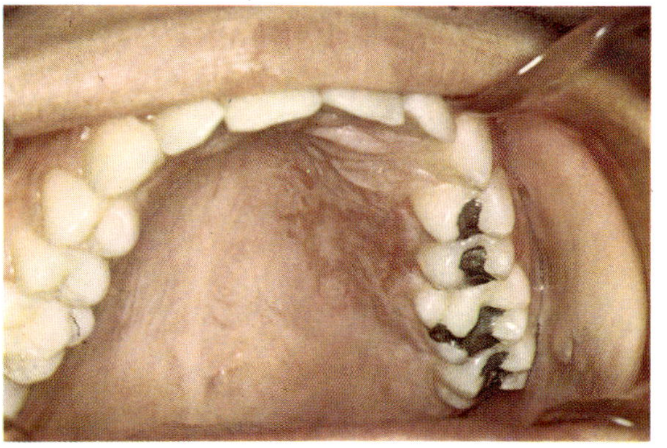

389 Herpes zoster The numerous vesicular and ulcerative lesions affecting the mucosa of the soft and hard palates are limited to the right side by the median palatal raphe in this pätient with herpes zoster. (See **40** and **289**)

389

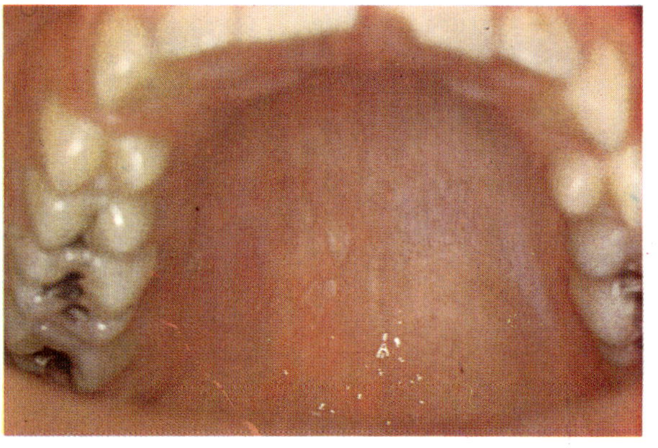

390 Herpangina The vesicular lesions affecting the soft palate and uvula in this child are due to infection by the Coxsackie virus.

390

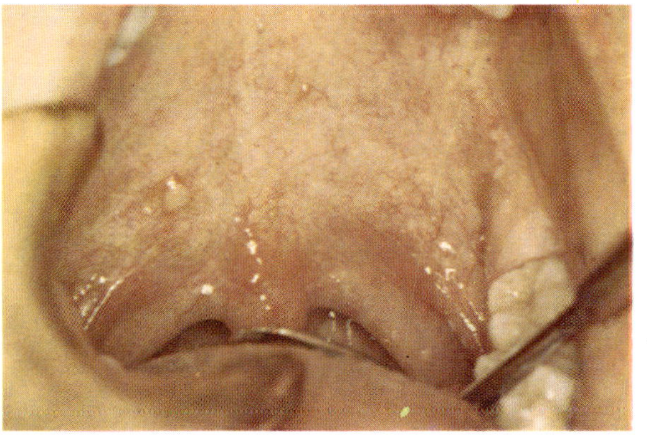

391 Denture sore mouth The bright red mucosa of the palate in this patient exactly delineates the area of tissue covered by a denture. Although such changes are frequently associated with chronic infection by Candida albicans, these organisms were not recoverable in culture from this area.

391

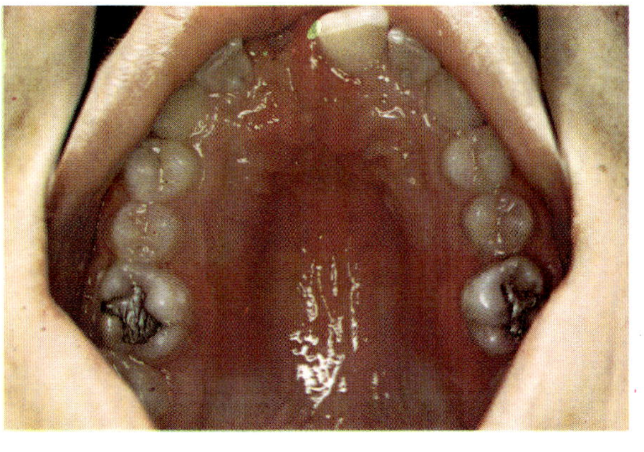

392 Acute pseudomembranous candidiasis (Thrush) The irregular white lesion covering the vault of the hard palate is due to infection with Candida albicans. The patient was receiving antibiotics and chemotherapy for leukaemia.

392

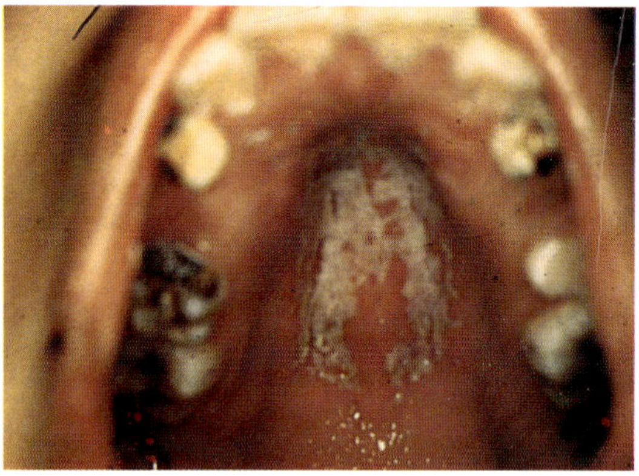

393 Ecchymosis of the soft palate This 9 year old girl presented with a fractured incisor and was noted at the same time to have an ecchymosis affecting the mucosa of the soft palate. No cause for the condition could be established.

393

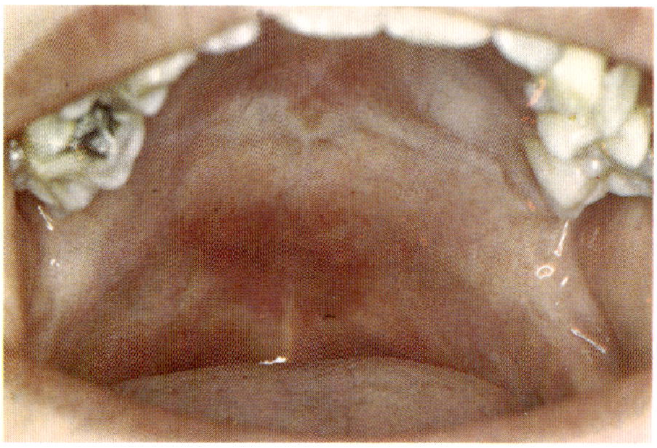

394 Leukaemia The black necrotic palatal mucosa adjacent to the maxillary central incisors in this 8 year old boy was the first indication of acute myelogenous leukaemia.

394

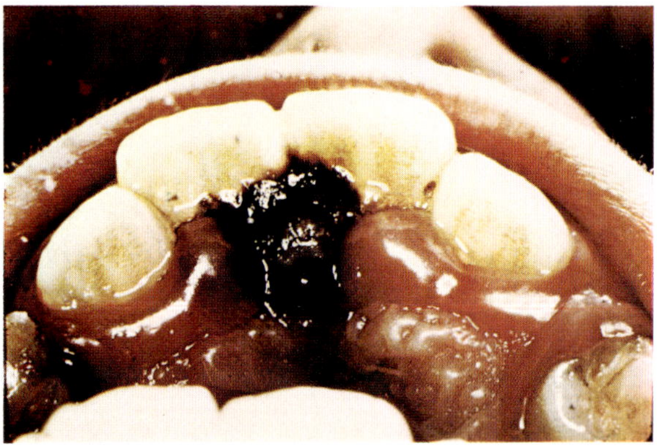

395 Rhabdomyosarcoma The bright red fungating lesion at the junction of the hard and soft palates in this 8 year old boy is a highly malignant recurrent rhabdomyosarcoma

395

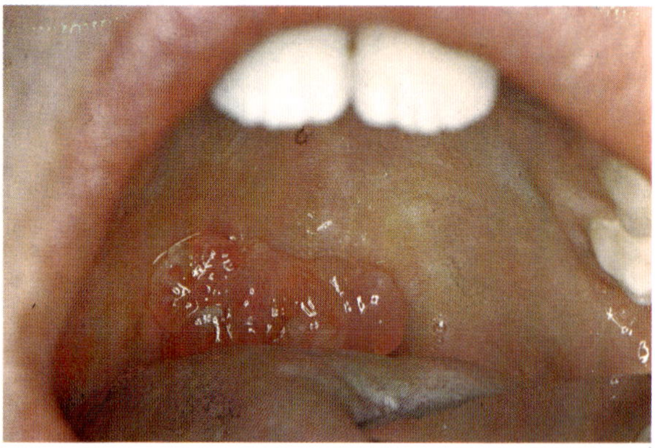

396 **Nasopalatine cyst** The inverted pear-shaped radiolucent lesion in the region of the incisive canal is evidence of a nasopalatine cyst.

396

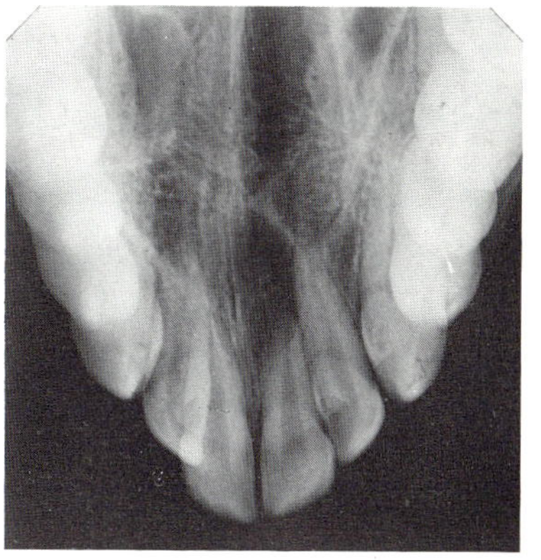

397 **Dentigerous cyst** This radiograph of the right maxillary incisor region shows an inverted mesiodens enveloped by a large radiolucent area. Biopsy confirmed the diagnosis of a dentigerous cyst. Note the extensive apical resorption of the central and lateral incisors.

397

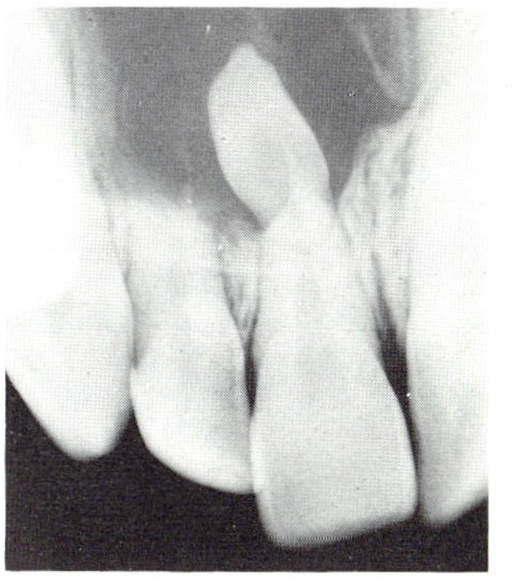

398 **Oedema of the uvula** The marked swelling of the uvula in this child is due to acute oedema. The cause was unknown.

398

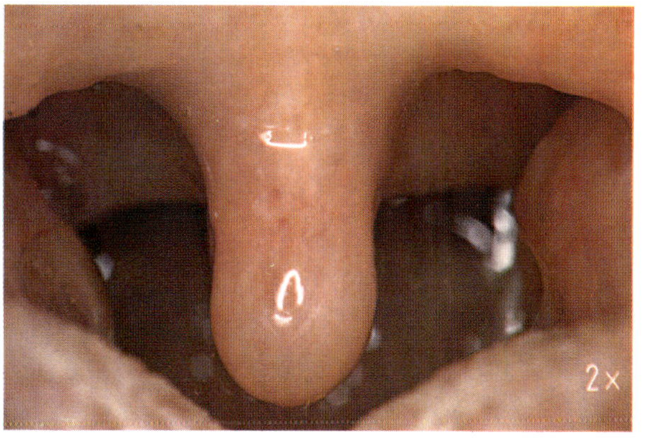

399 **Tonsillar enlargement** Enlargement of the tonsils in this child with hyperthyroidism is so gross that the tissues almost meet in the midline.

399

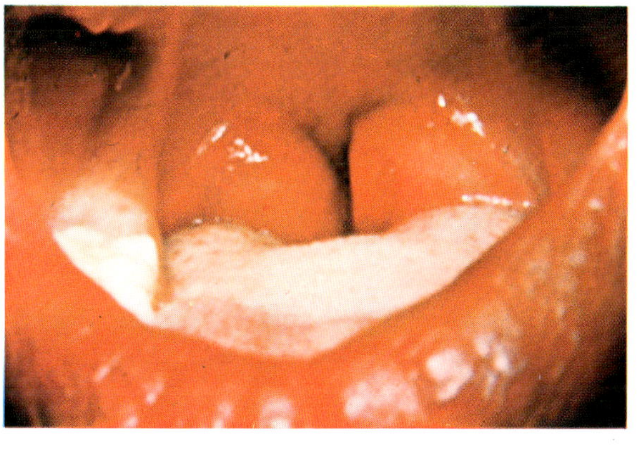

6. The tongue

400 Macroglossia Although tongue enlargement, or macroglossia, has produced most of the lingual protrusion in this 3 year old boy, there is also a functional element, in that it is necessary for him to protrude his tongue in order to breathe through his mouth. His nasal airway is obstructed by grossly enlarged tonsils and adenoids.

400

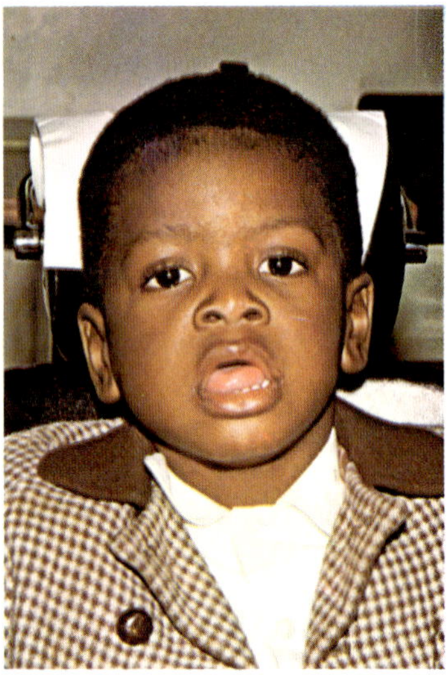

401 Tongue thrust This child's tongue is thrust between the incisor teeth in swallowing and remains in contact with the lower lip at rest. The abnormal tongue activity is associated with an incomplete incisal overbite (anterior open bite).

401

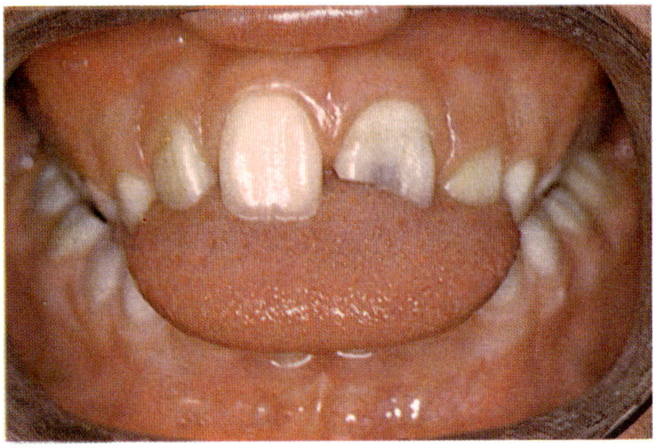

402 Lymphangioma The congenital enlargement of the tongue in this young child is caused by the presence of a lymphangioma composed of numerous lymph vessels and spaces.

402

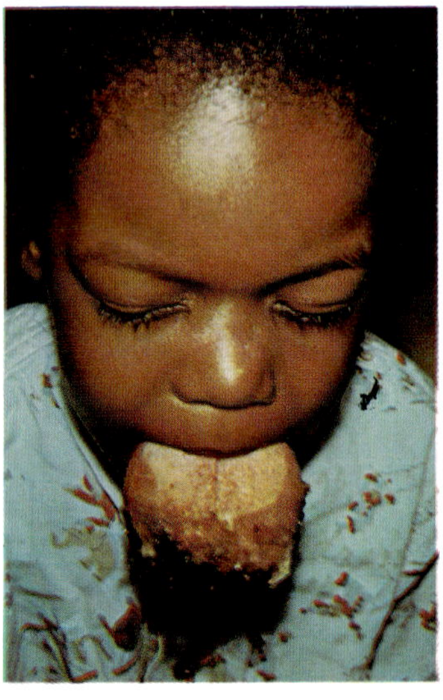

403 Lymphangioma The lump on the side of the tongue in this 6 year old girl has been present for nearly three years. It started as a small 'blister' and gradually increased in size. The lesion is soft and on transillumination appears to consist of a number of fluid-filled spaces. Excision biopsy confirmed a diagnosis of lymphangioma.

403

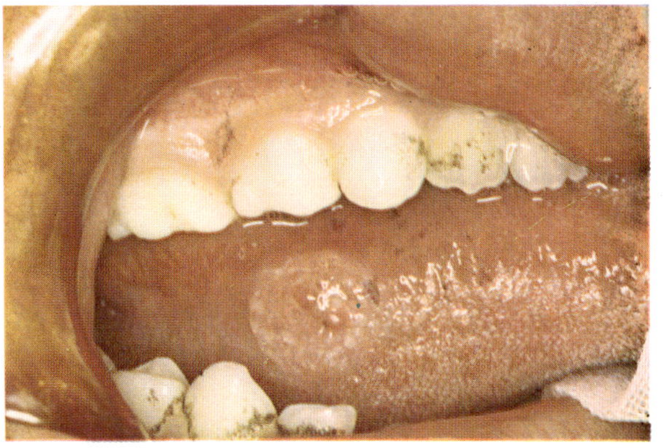

404 Haematoma This haemophiliac patient, as a result of biting his tongue, has developed a severe and large haematoma.

404

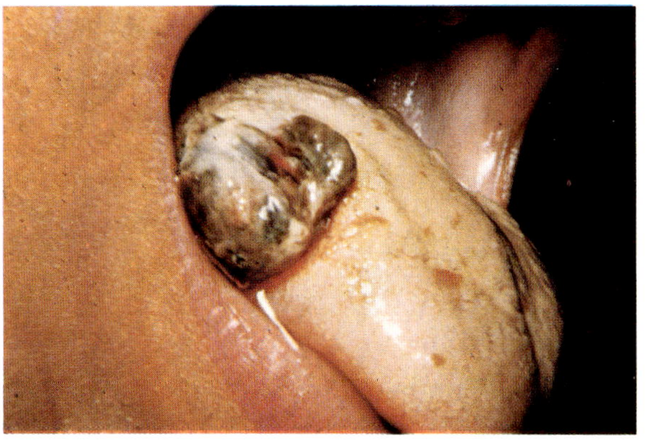

405 Median rhomboid glossitis The circumscribed smooth area of depapillation in the midline of the tongue immediately anterior to the foramen caecum is characteristic of the condition known as median rhomboid glossitis.

405

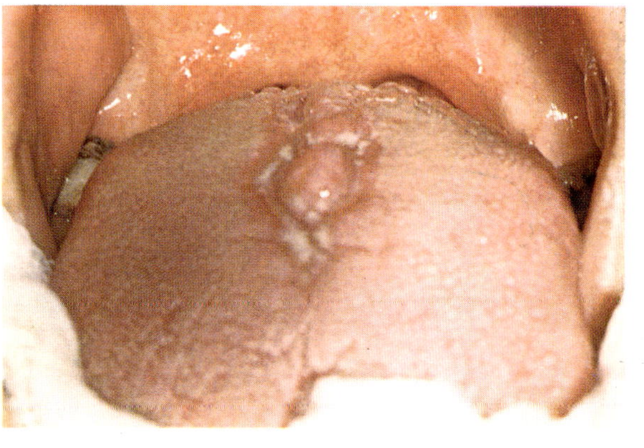

406 Popsicle (Ice-lolly) tongue A large area of hyperkeratosis on the dorsal surface of this child's tongue formed in response to irritation from the frequent eating of popsicles, or ice lollies.

406

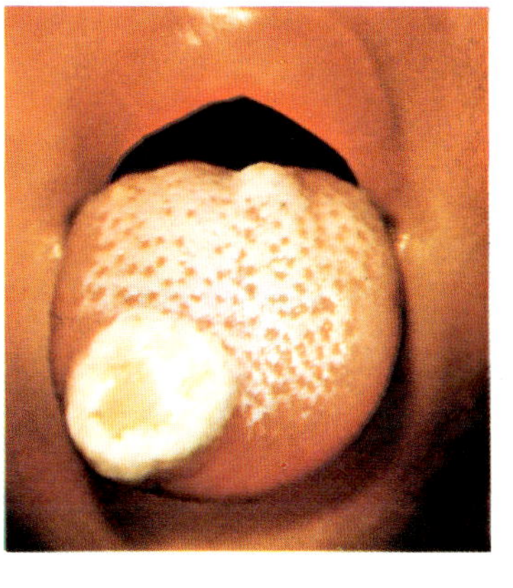

407 Fibroepithelial polyp The pedunculated lesion on the central aspect of the tongue in this 13 year old girl measured approximately 6mm in diameter. No cause could be established for this 'fibroepithelial' polyp which regressed spontaneously in about 2 months.

407

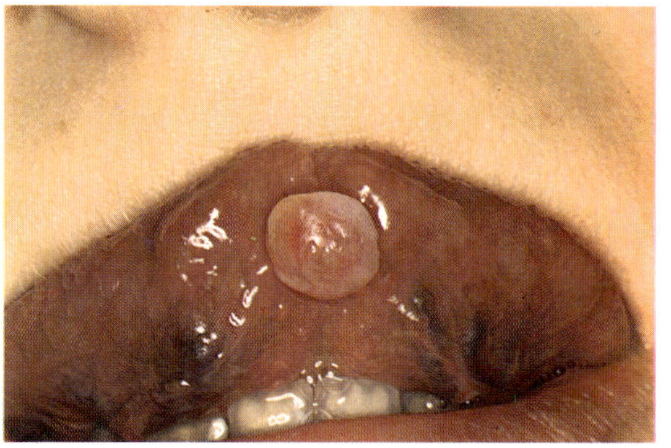

408 Mucocele The lesion at the tip of the tongue in this $7\frac{1}{2}$ year old girl had been present for 6 weeks. Excision biopsy confirmed the diagnosis of a mucous extravasation cyst.

408

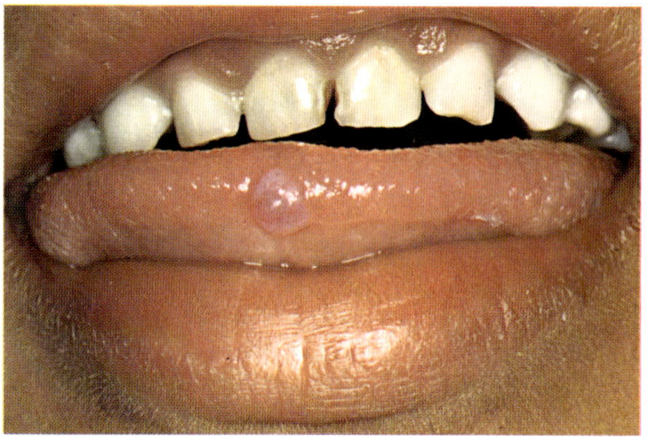

409 Papilloma The small pedunculated lesion with finger-like processes on the lateral aspect of the tongue of a girl aged 10 years is a papilloma.

409

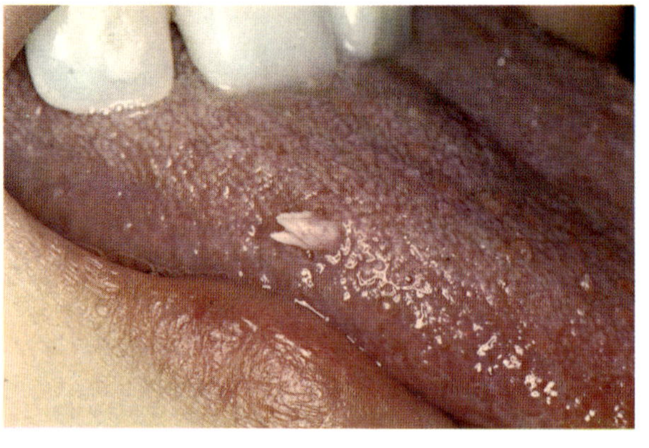

410, 411 Orodigitofacial dysostosis (OFD syndrome) The lobulated tongues of two members of a family with the OFD syndrome are characteristic for this X-linked dominant genetic defect. Note the whitish hamartomata present between the lobules on the tip of the tongue. (See **366** and **472**)

410

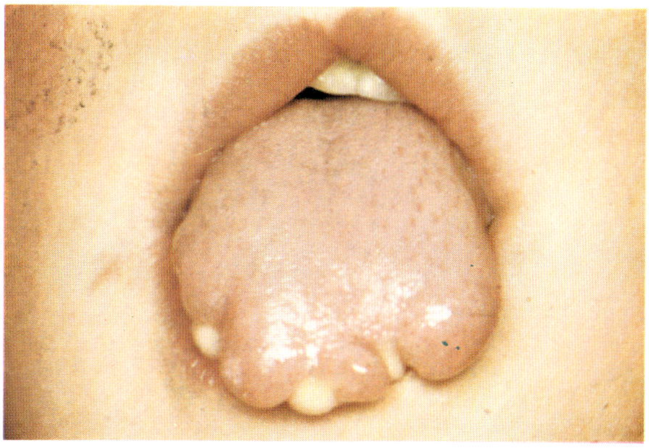

411

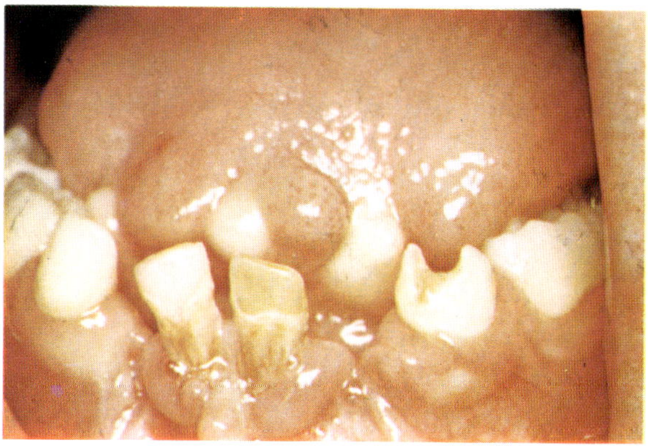

412 Electrical burn of tongue The scarring and deformity of the tongue were caused by an electrical burn at the age of 3 years. (See **382**)

412

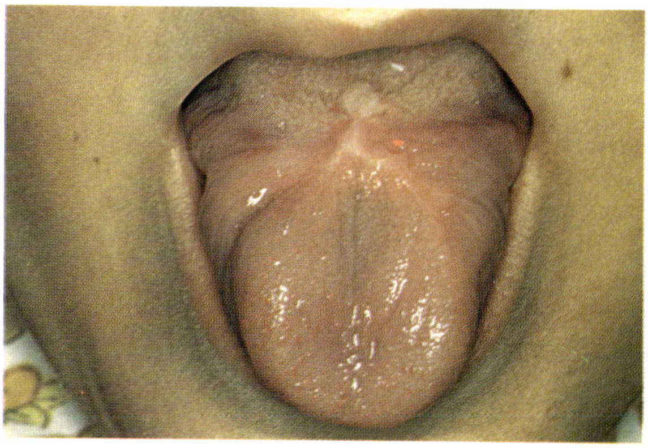

413 Geographic tongue The dorsum of the tongue in this child shows irregular areas which lack filiform papillae, leaving a reddish smooth surface. These areas tend to migrate anteriorly and laterally. The condition is generally asymptomatic in children.

413

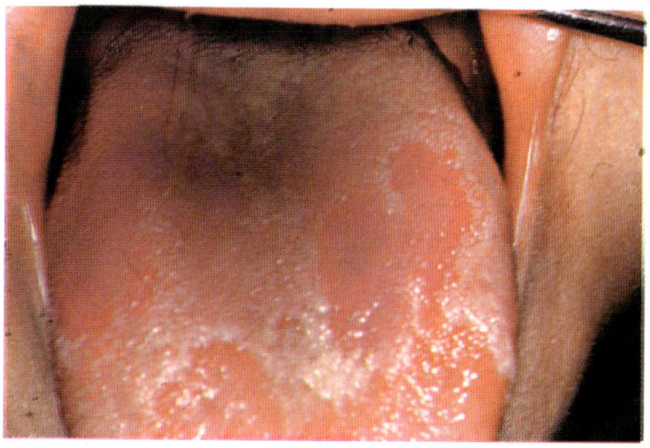

414

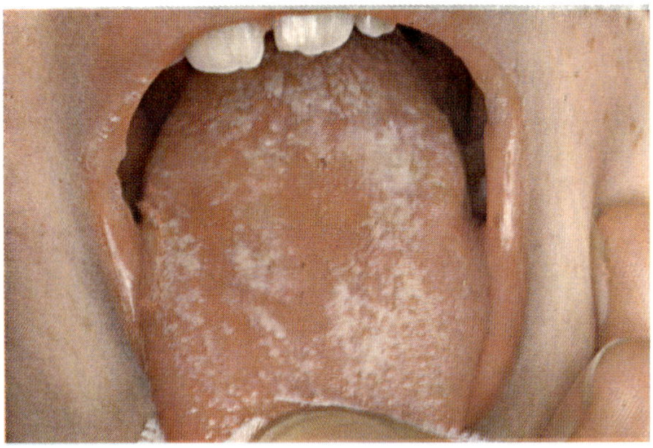

414 Acute pseudomembranous candidiasis (Thrush) The dorsum of the tongue in this 10 year old boy is diffusely covered by the white plaques which form part of a generalised acute candidal stomatitis.

415

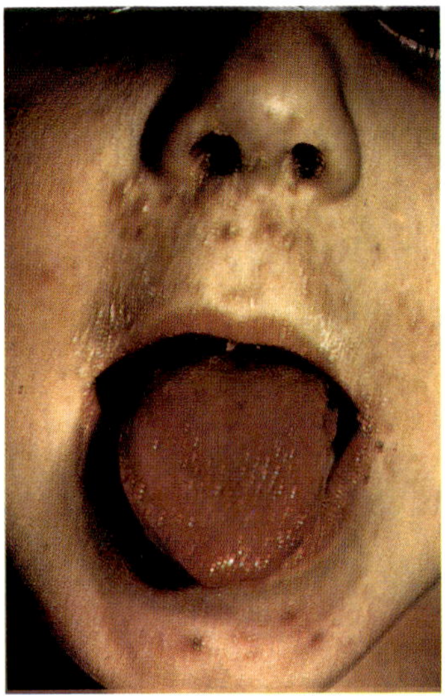

415 Raspberry (Red strawberry) tongue of scarlet fever In the early stages of scarlet fever the tongue becomes coated with a white fur through which the fungiform papillae project (white strawberry tongue). By the fourth day desquamation occurs and the dorsum of the tongue, as seen in this child, is left bright red with prominent papillae – the red strawberry or raspberry tongue.

416

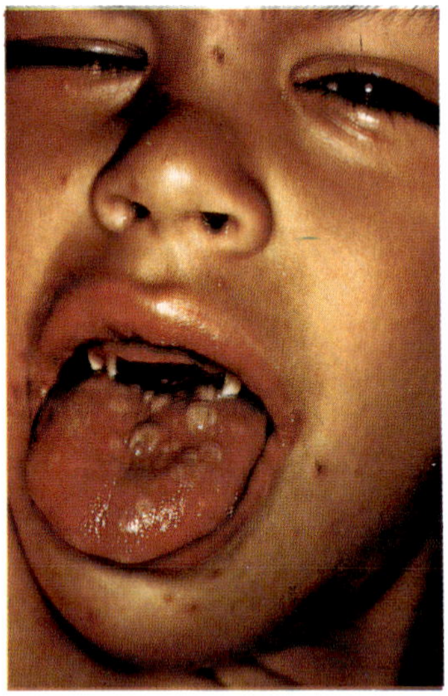

416 Chicken pox (Varicella) The tongue is frequently involved during the onset of the viral disease chicken pox. This child shows the typical vesicles, some of which have already ruptured to form painful ulcers covered by a white or yellowish exudate.

417 Acute herpetic gingivostomatitis This 9 year old girl presented with an extremely sore mouth. Scattered over the dorsum of the tongue are the typical herpetic ulcers with a yellowish centre and a surrounding erythematous halo.

417

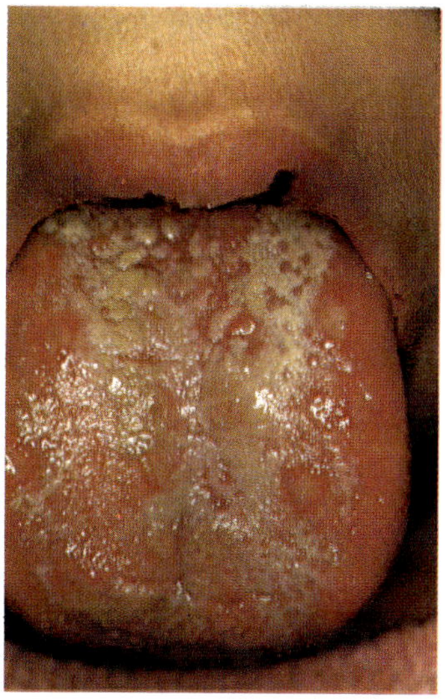

418 Staphylococcal ulceration The curious ulceration of the tissues at the tip of the tongue in this child is covered by a characteristic bright yellow slough. Bacteriological culture from the lesion produced a pure growth of coagulase positive Staphylococcus aureus.

418

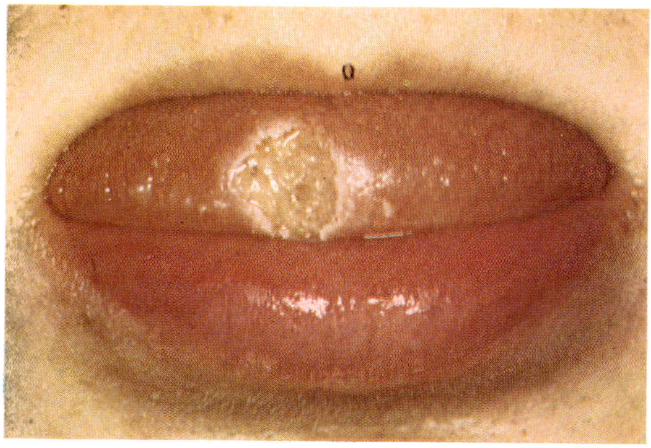

419 Recurrent aphthous ulceration The deeply punched out aphthous ulcer on the lateral aspect of the tongue in this girl was extremely painful and had been present for more than a week. This lesion is typical of the major variety of aphthae and is usually associated with similar lesions on other non-keratinised mucosal surfaces. (See **334**)

419

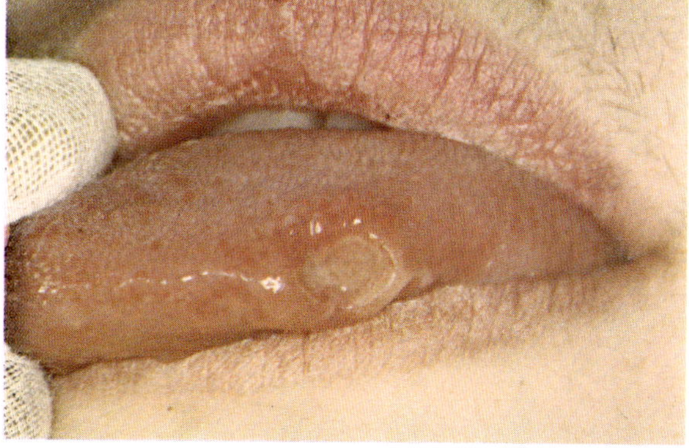

420

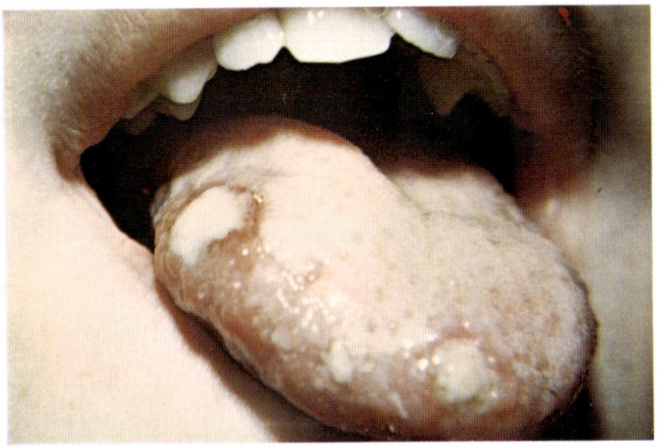

420 Periodic (Cyclic) neutropenia Two irregular ulcers are present on the dorsum of the tongue in this child suffering from periodic neutropenia. (See **297**)

421

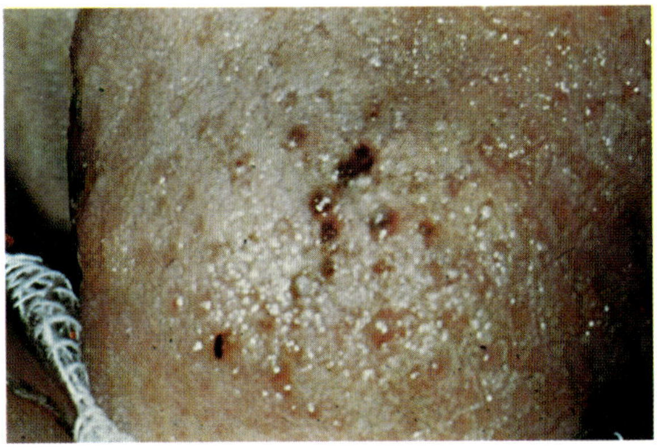

421 Aplastic anaemia Superimposed on the extremely pallid mucosa of the tongue in this child with aplastic anaemia is a crop of discrete petechial haemorrhages due to an associated thrombocytopenia.

422

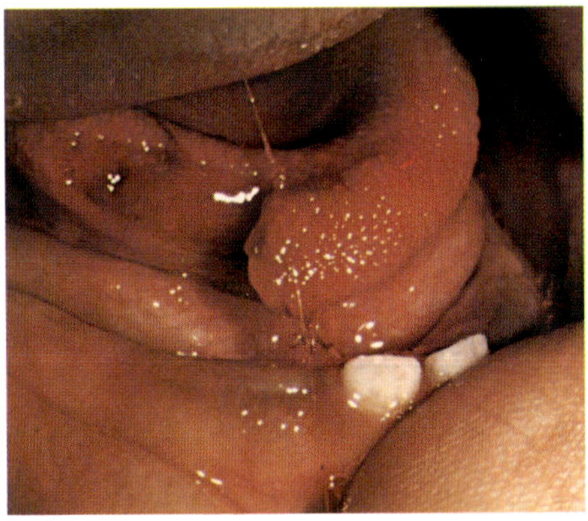

422 Laceration of tongue The severe laceration of the tongue in this infant was due to perforation by the incisor teeth from indirect trauma on the underside of the chin.

423

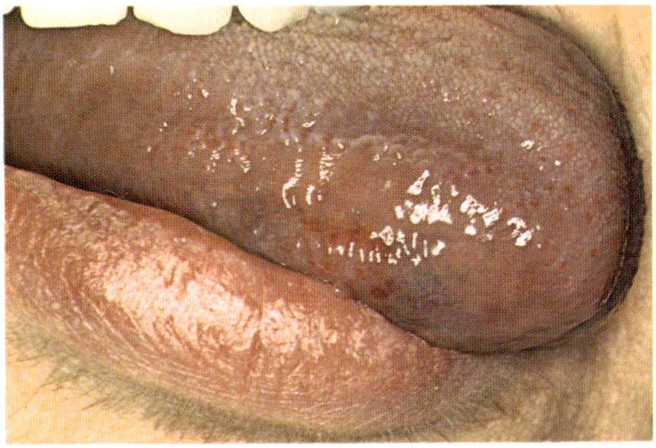

423 Abrasion of tongue Immediately after regional (block) anaesthesia of the inferior dental nerve, this patient bit the lateral aspect of the tongue producing a superficial abrasion and bruising of the tissues.

7. *The jaws*

a. Maxilla

424 Anodontia The only teeth present in the jaws of this young boy are two erupted mandibular second primary molars; there is anodontia of the permanent dentition. The lateral skull radiograph illustrates the complete failure of maxillary alveolar development seen in such cases.

424

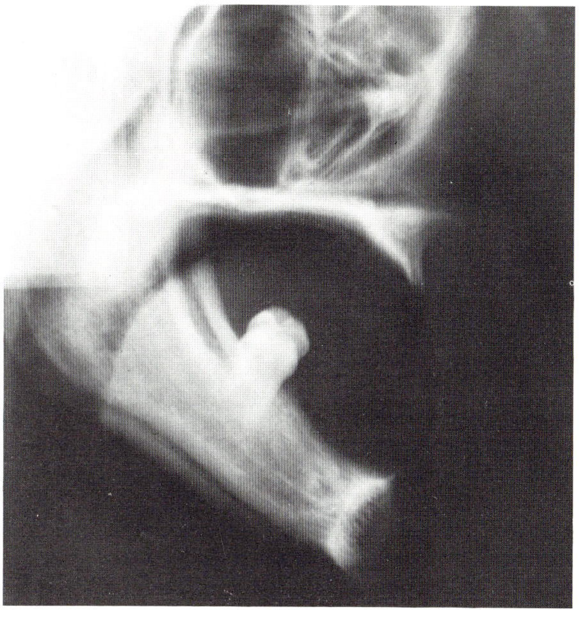

425

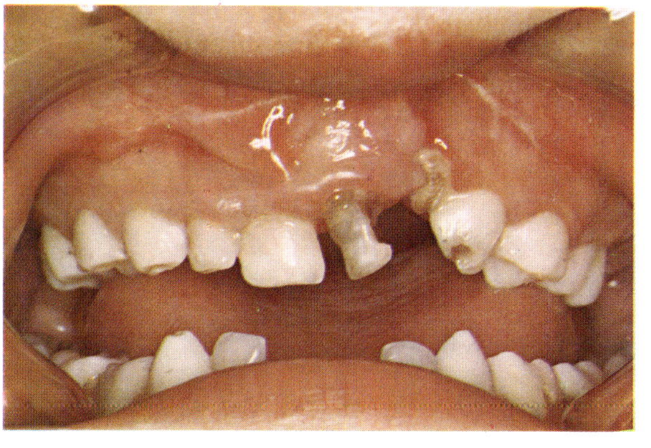

425 Cleft lip and palate The unilateral cleft lip and palate in this girl had been repaired in infancy leaving her with a persistent oro-nasal fistula through the anterior portions of the hard palate. The maxillary left lateral incisors in the primary and permanent dentitions are missing and a supernumerary 'pre-canine' is present distal to the cleft. As is common in children with clefts, plaque deposition is responsible for gross carious destruction of the primary teeth adjacent to the defect. (See **42** and **43**)

426

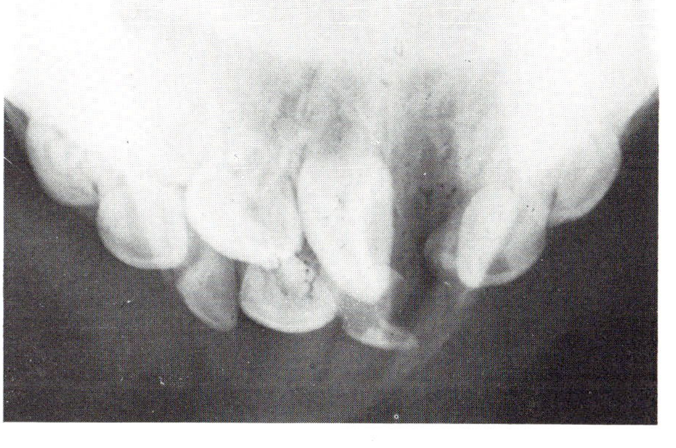

426 Radiograph of the case seen in **425**.

427 Cleft lip and palate Anomalous tooth development is common in association with clefts of the maxillary alveolus. A supernumerary 'pre-canine' is present in both the primary and permanent dentitions.

427

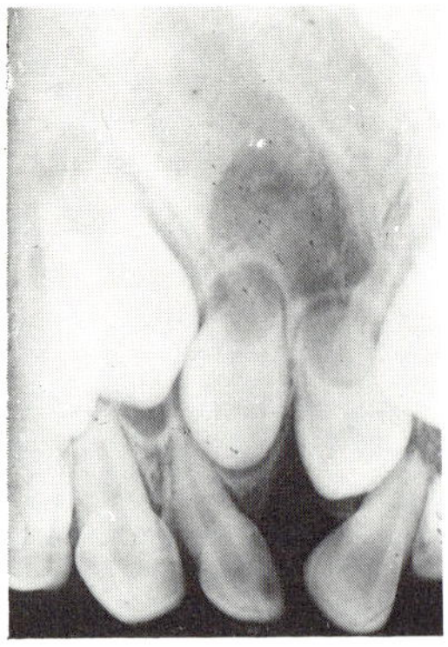

428 Globulomaxillary cyst The well-defined area of bony rarefaction lying between the maxillary right permanent lateral incisor and canine is evidence of a cystic lesion. The cyst is displacing the roots of the adjacent teeth, both of which responded normally to vitality tests. As doubt has recently been cast on the existence of fissural cysts in this region, the possible diagnosis of a lateral periodontal cyst can not be excluded.

428

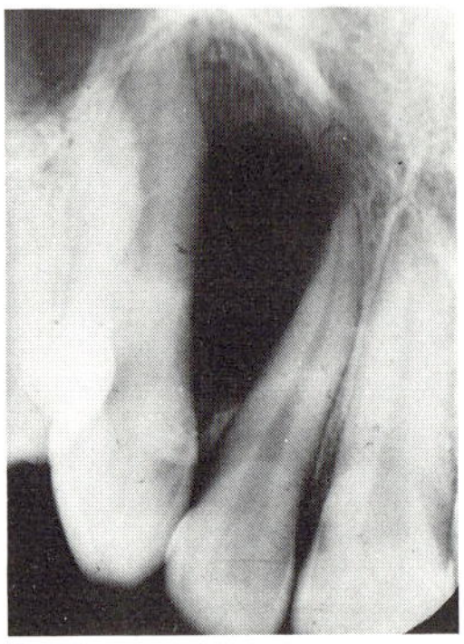

429, 430 Periodontal abscess These 2 radiographs of the maxillary incisor region from a 16 year old girl were taken before and after treatment. Note the approximation of the roots of the incisor teeth once the pressure from the suppurative lesion was removed. Both incisors were vital and the palatal access cavities had been made in error by the referring dentist. A differential diagnosis of infected lateral periodontal cyst is possible in this case; the source of the infection was never established.

429

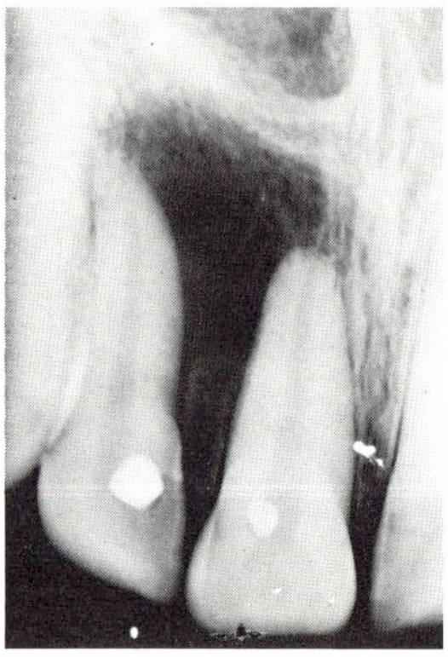

430

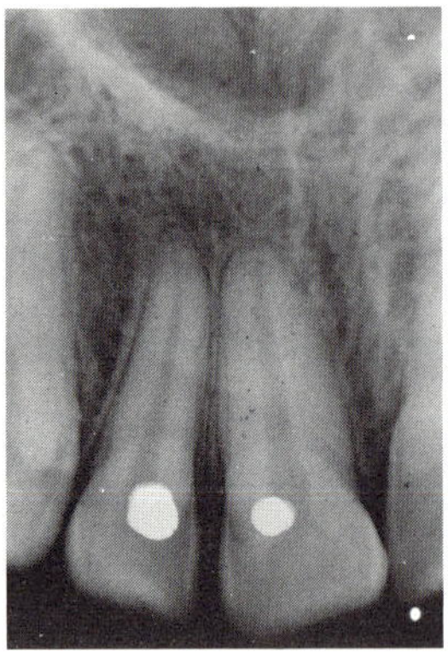

431 Eruption cyst A bluish, fluctuant swelling overlying the unerupted maxillary right permanent canine was noted in this 10 year old boy. Marsupialisation of the eruption cyst resulted in rapid emergence of the tooth.

431

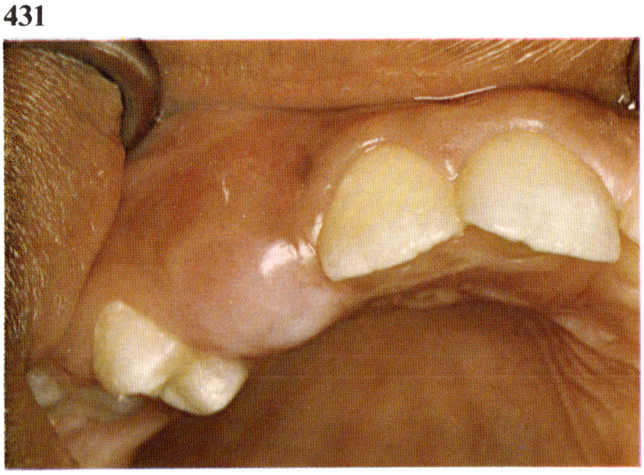

432 Melanotic neuroectodermal tumour of infancy An occlusal radiograph of an infant with swelling of the left maxilla shows a destructive bony lesion in the region of the central incisor which is labially displaced. Excision biopsy confirmed the diagnosis of melanotic neuroectodermal tumour of infancy.

432

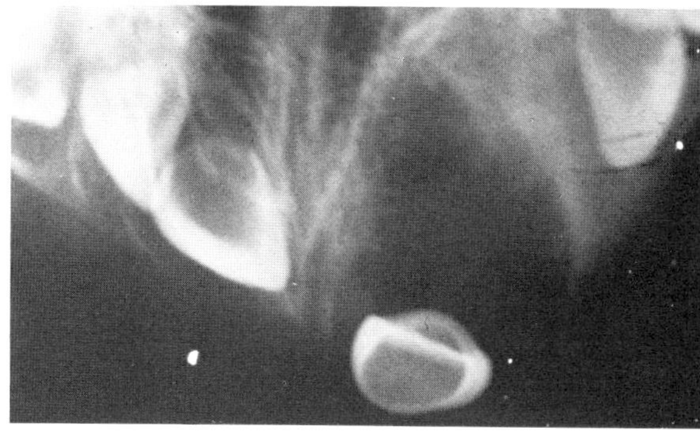

433 Dentigerous cyst This radiograph shows a large area of bony rarefaction surrounding the crown of the unerupted and displaced maxillary permanent lateral incisor. The lesion is a dentigerous cyst which appears to be associated with the retained and non-vital primary lateral incisor.

433

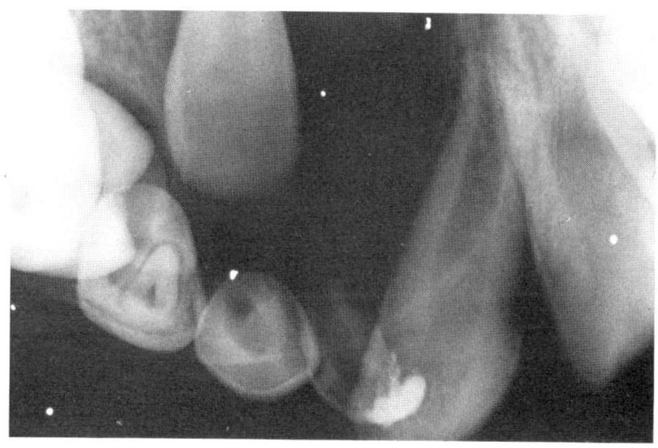

434 Ameloblastic fibro-odontoma Delayed eruption of the maxillary left permanent central incisor is associated with a rarefying lesion of alveolar bone within which is seen an area of calcification. Excision biopsy showed the tumour to be an example of a rare ameloblastic fibro-odontoma.

434

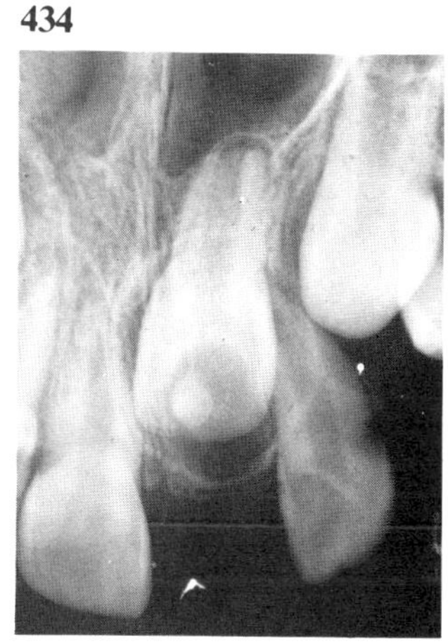

435 Compound odontome The maxillary permanent right central and lateral incisors had failed to erupt in this 10 year old child.

435

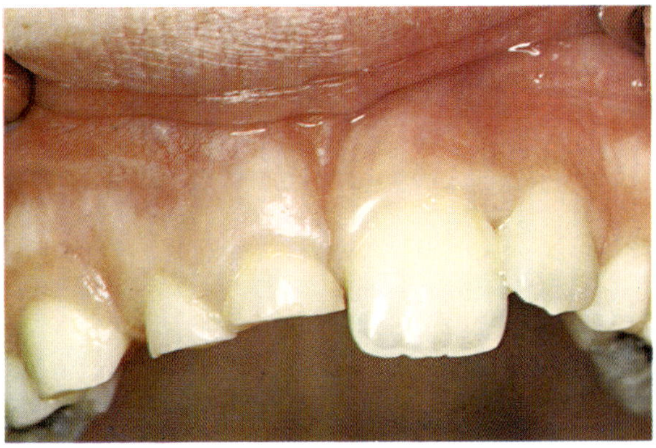

436 A radiograph of the region seen in **435** shows a large irregular calcified mass displacing the permanent incisors distally. Surgical removal of the lesion showed it to be composed of a number of separate denticles.

436

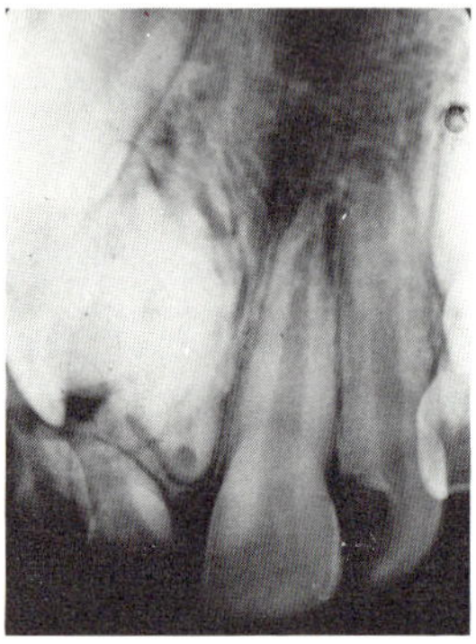

437 Fibrous dysplasia Enlargement on the left side of the maxilla in this teenage girl is associated with ectopic eruption of the left permanent central incisor and retention of the primary central incisor.

437

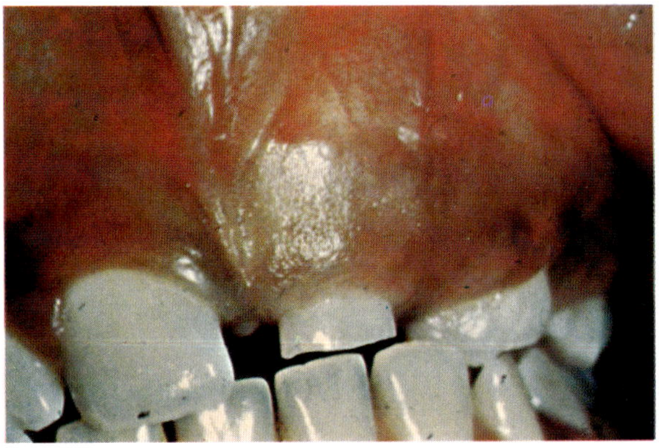

438 An occlusal radiograph of the affected area seen in **437** shows the typical 'ground-glass' appearance of the bone seen in fibrous dysplasia.

438

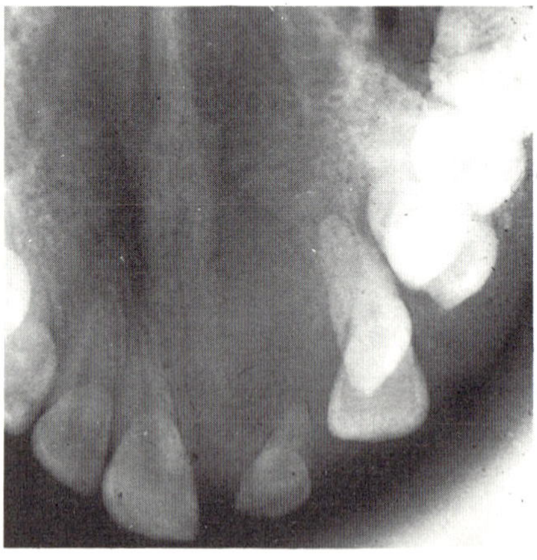

439

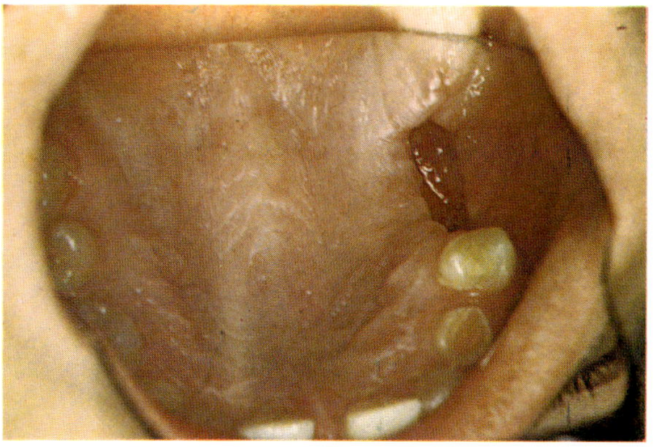

439 Histiocytosis X (Hand-Schüller-Christian type) This 14 year old boy presented with a history of diabetes insipidus and many mobile teeth. The necrotic tissue underlying the maxillary left second premolar and first molar may be seen after tooth removal. Biopsy of the involved tissues confirmed the diagnosis of Histiocytosis X – Hand-Schüller-Christian type. (See **365**)

440

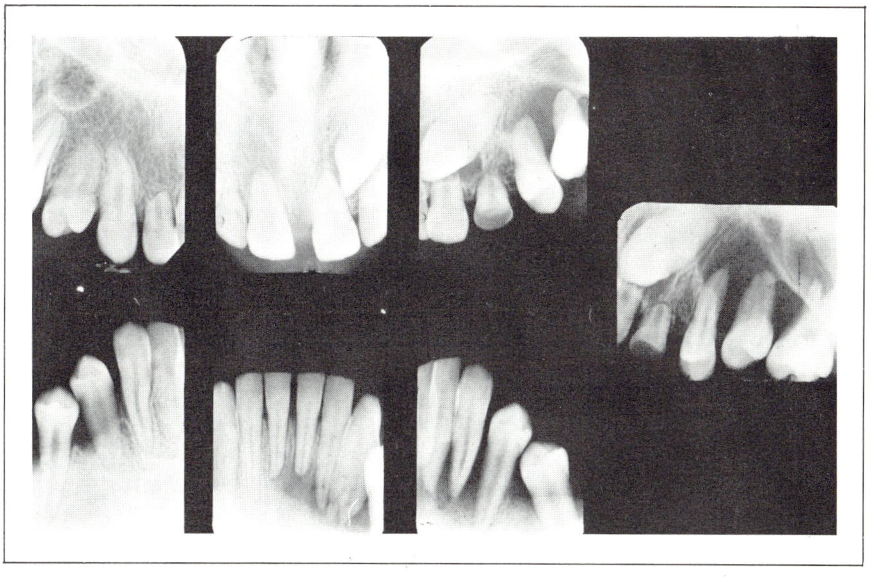

440 Radiographs of the case seen in **439** show bilateral lesions with bony rarefaction in the mandible and in the left maxilla.

441

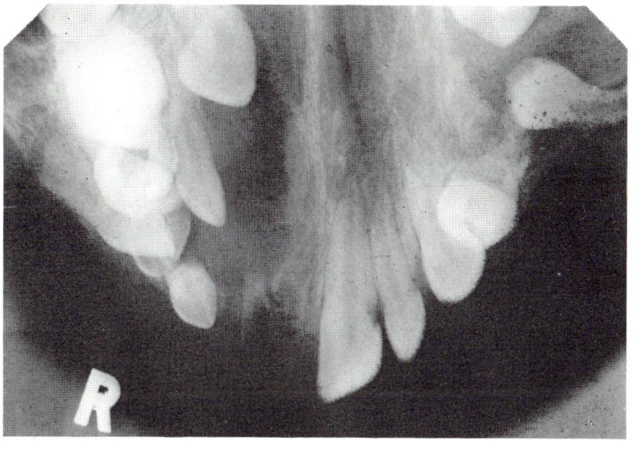

441 Multiple dentigerous cysts This radiograph of a 9 year old girl reveals two dentigerous cysts of the maxilla; one large cyst involves the unerupted lateral incisor on the right side of the jaw with displacement of the central incisor, canine and first premolar; the other involves the unerupted left second premolar. On both sides the cysts are associated with non-vital and retained primary teeth, on the right the lateral incisor and on the left the second molar. There is no evidence to support a diagnosis of Gorlin's syndrome in this case.

442 Dentigerous cyst A dentigerous cyst was present in an 18 year old male patient and involved a palatally placed mesiodens. Histological examination of the cyst lining showed the presence of non-keratinised squamous cell epithelium with goblet cell metaplasia.

442

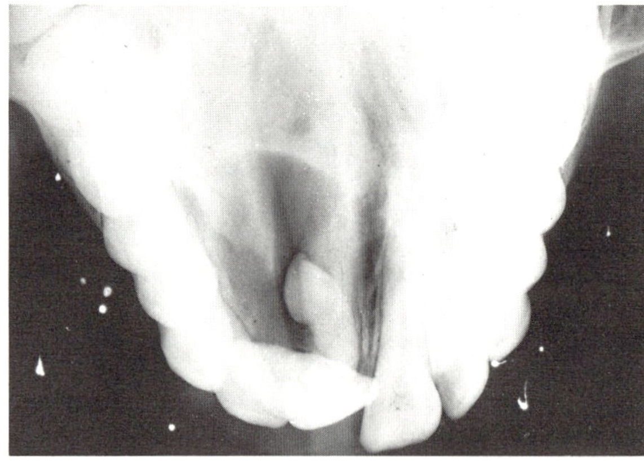

443 Radicular cyst A very large maxillary cystic lesion is seen in this radiograph from a 13 year old boy. The lesion derives from an apical cyst on a fractured and non-vital left central incisor which had remained untreated for 4 years.

443

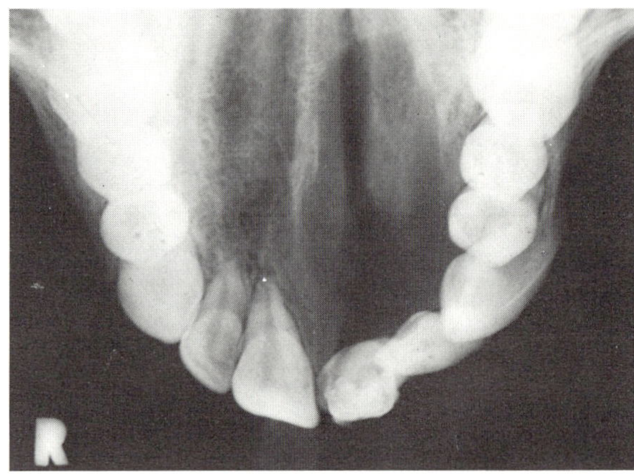

b. Mandible

444 Malposition of tooth germ The developing second premolar in this 4 year old girl is mesially displaced from its normal position between the roots of the second primary molar.

444

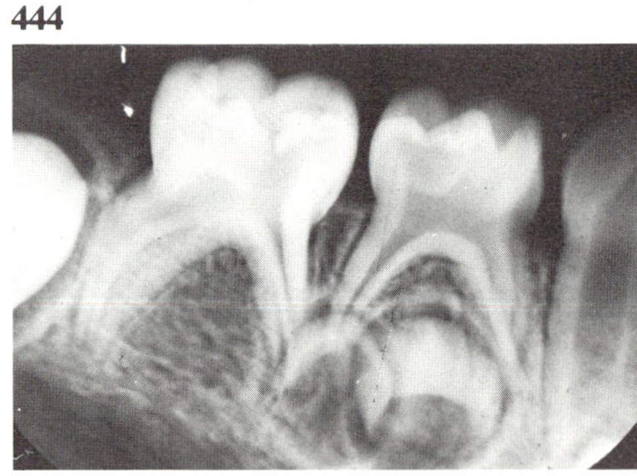

445 Osteomyelitis Bony sequestration of a portion of the left mandible in a 4 year old boy with osteomyelitis.

445

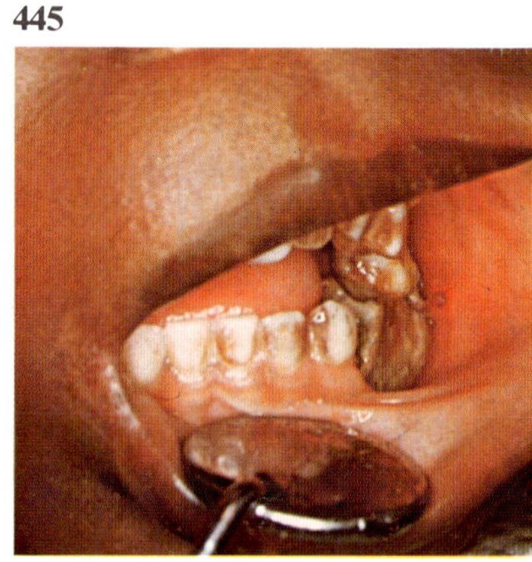

446

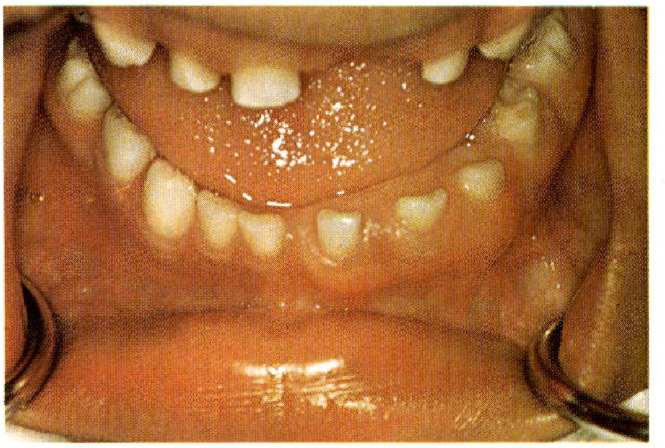

446 Fibrous dysplasia The enlargement of the mandibular alveolar process extending from the left primary canine to the midline in this young child is due to fibrous dysplasia.

447

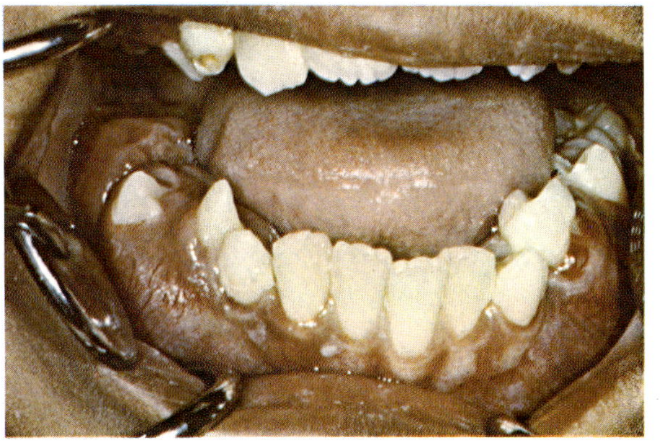

447 Burkitt's lymphoma This 11 year old boy recently noticed swelling of his gums, followed by pain and loosening of his teeth. All the teeth in the mandible were loose, as were teeth on the right side of the maxilla.

448

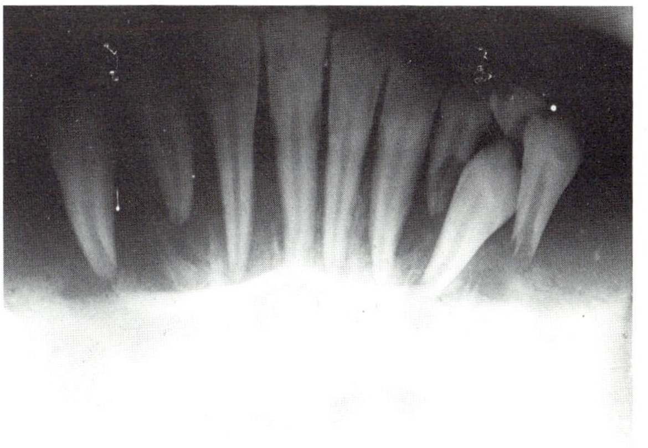

448 A radiograph of the patient seen in **447** shows the gross destructive changes in bone around all the erupted mandibular teeth. Biopsy from the mandible confirmed the diagnosis of Burkitt's lymphoma.

449

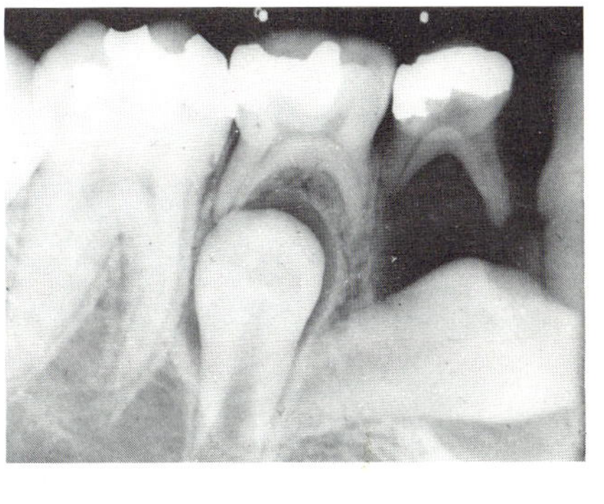

449 Dentigerous cyst The extensive area of bony rarefaction involving the periradicular tissues of the first primary molar and the crown of the unerupted first premolar, together with the displacement of the latter tooth, is diagnostic of a dentigerous cyst.

450 Ameloblastoma The large area of bony rarefaction involving the unerupted mandibular first permanent molar and distal root of the second primary molar which is pathologically resorbed, proved to be due to the presence of an ameloblastoma. Note the well circumscribed bony outline of the lesion.

450

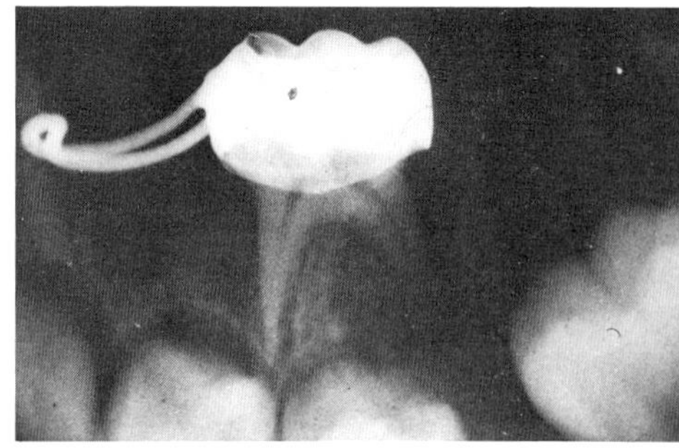

451, 452 Complex odontome The irregularly calcified mass in the right mandibular incisor region is the calcified portion of a complex odontome in an 8 year old boy who presented with considerable bony enlargement of the jaw. The adjacent area of rarefaction, with thinning of the cortical plate, although 'cystic' in appearance is caused by the soft tissue component of the odontome.

451

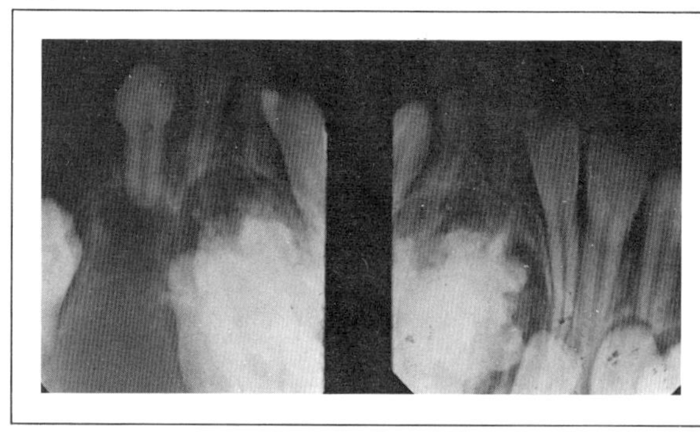

452

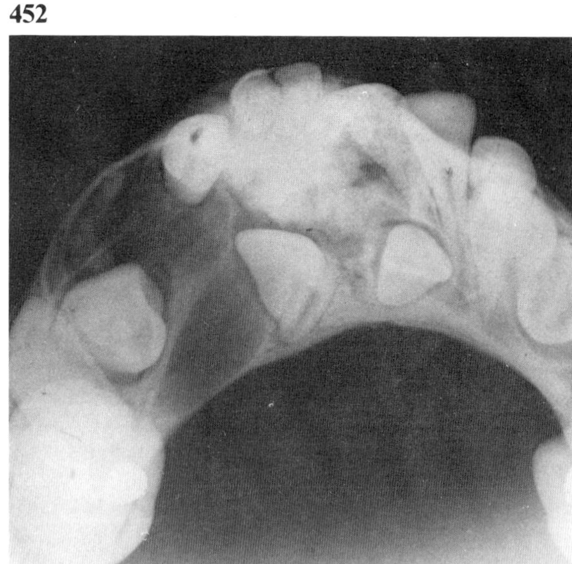

453, 454 Cementifying fibroma The large area of rarefaction and swelling of the right mandible seen in the radiographs of this 9 year old boy proved after excision and biopsy to be due to a cementifying fibroma. Note the distortion and thinning of the lower and lateral borders of the mandible and the considerable displacement of the second premolar tooth germ caused by this tumour.

453

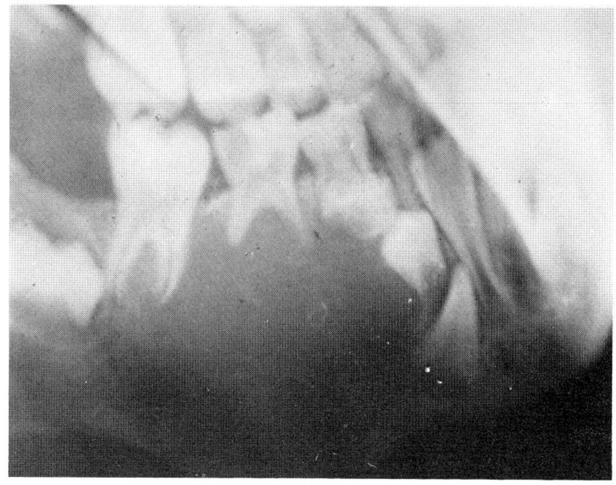

454

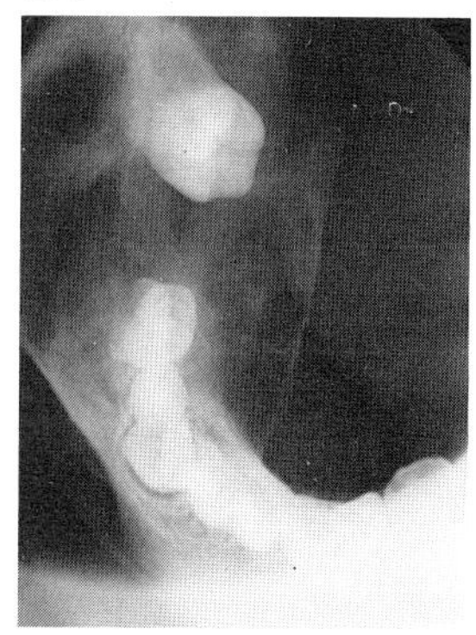

455 Haemorrhagic (Traumatic, solitary) bone cyst The poorly defined area of rarefaction in the body of the left mandible subjacent to the second permanent molar is caused by a haemorrhagic bone cyst. There is no associated jaw swelling and the adjacent teeth are all vital.

455

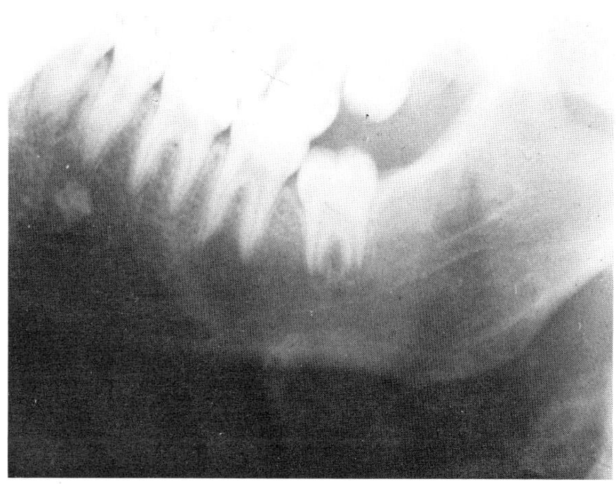

456

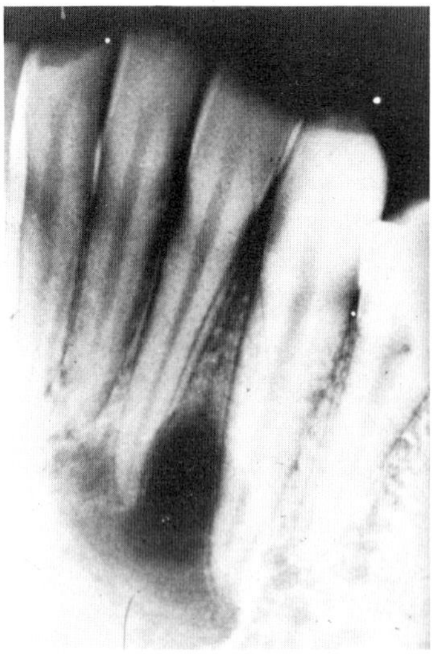

456 Haemorrhagic (Traumatic, solitary) bone cyst
The area of bony rarefaction lying between the apical portions of the roots of the permanent left lateral incisor and canine is due to a haemorrhagic bone cyst. Note the continued presence of the lamina dura around the roots of the adjacent teeth, both of which are vital.

457

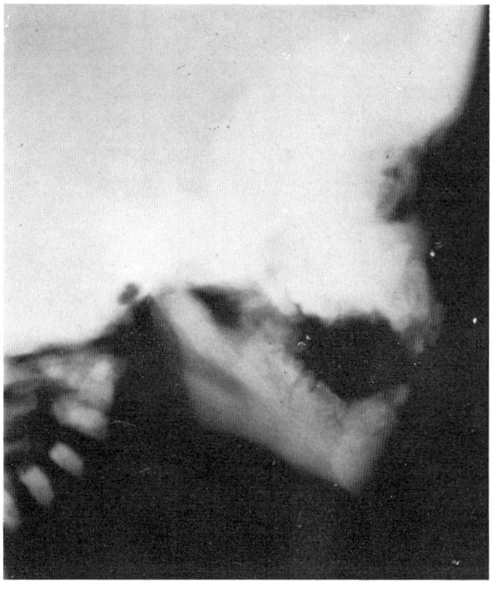

458

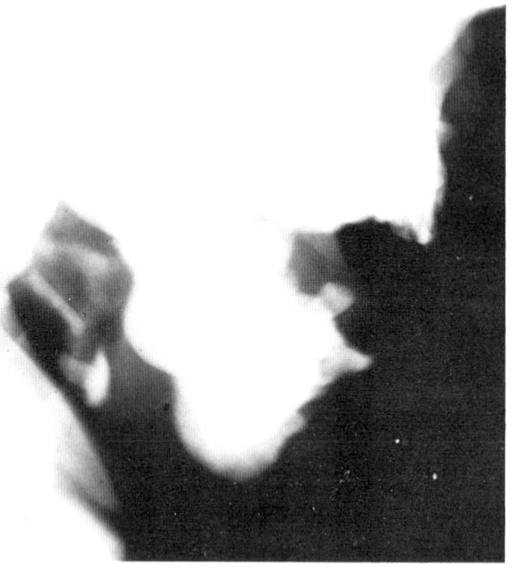

457, 458 Osteopetrosis (Albers-Schönberg disease)
Two radiographs of an 8 year old boy with osteopetrosis showing the increased density of bones in this condition. The excessive bone deposition beneath the anterior portions of the horizontal ramus of the mandible in the second film is in response to chronic osteomyelitis of the jaw – a frequent complication. Delay in, or failure of, eruption of teeth is another feature of this condition.

8. *The limbs*

The illustrations in this chapter have been included as they either complete a clinical picture of, or are closely related to, conditions already described in the Atlas.

a. Upper limb

459 Arachnodactyly (Marfan's syndrome) The long tapering 'spider' fingers of arachnodactyly are seen in this child with Marfan's syndrome. Clubbing of the terminal phalanges is also frequently seen in association with this syndrome. (See **380**)

459

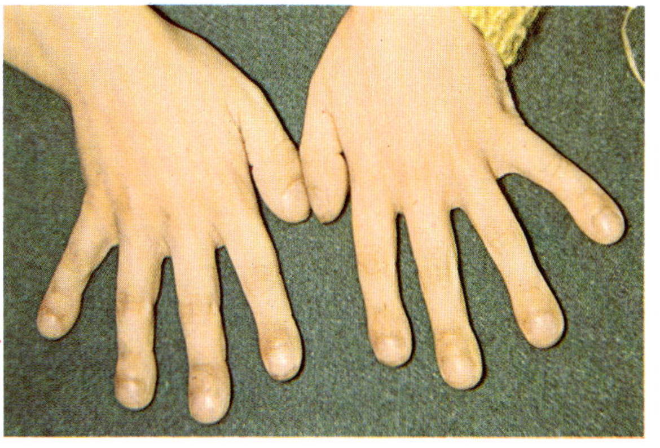

460 Syndactyly Complete fusion of the middle and ring fingers of both hands are present in this patient with syndactyly.

460

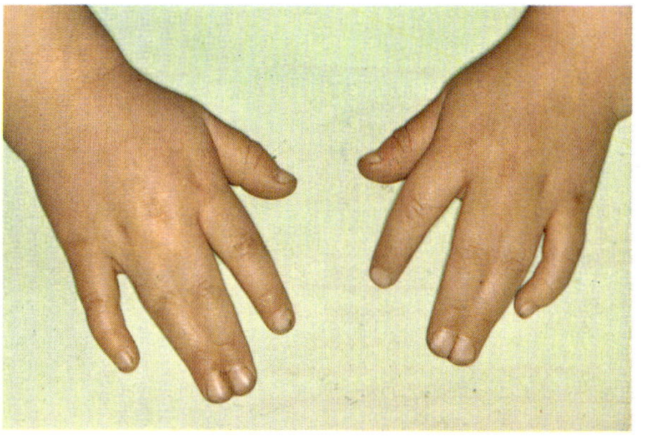

461 Orodigitofacial dysostosis (OFD syndrome) Webbing of ring and fifth fingers is evidence of partial syndactyly in this child with the OFD syndrome. Other abnormalities of the fingers and toes seen in this syndrome include polydactyly and clinodactyly. (See **366**, **410** and **411**)

461

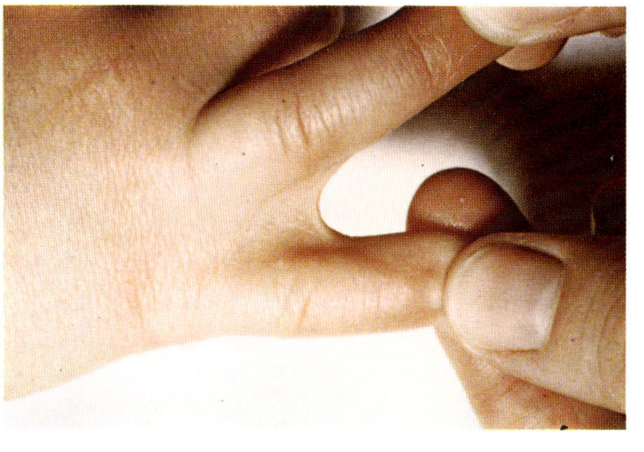

462

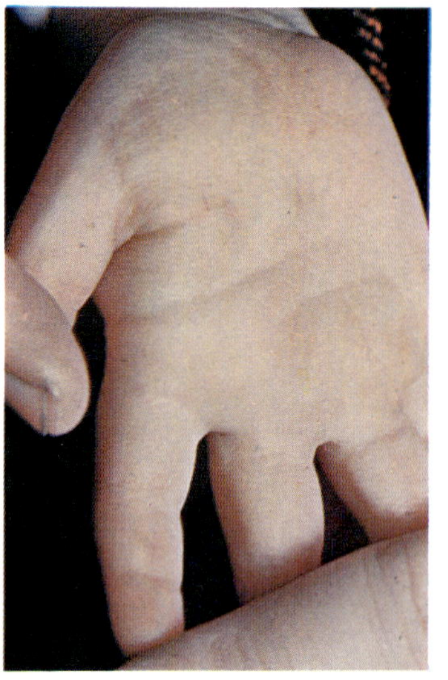

462 Papillon-Lefèvre syndrome (Hyperkeratosis palmoplantaris with periodontosis) Hyperkeratotic lesions affecting the palmar skin of this 3 year old girl are a characteristic component of the Papillon-Lefèvre syndrome. Similar lesions were present on the plantar surfaces of the feet and these changes were associated with severe periodontal tissue destruction in the primary dentition. (See **213** and **214**)

463

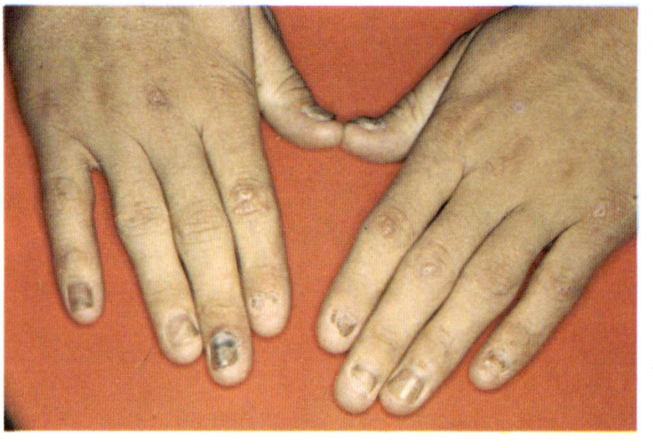

463 Epidermolysis bullosa dystrophica The dystrophic changes in the nails and the 'tissue paper' scars to the skin overlying the metacarpal-phalangeal and interphalangeal joints are residual signs of epidermolysis bullosa dystrophica in this adolescent boy. This is probably a mild case of the autosomal recessive variety of this abnormality. (See **167**)

464

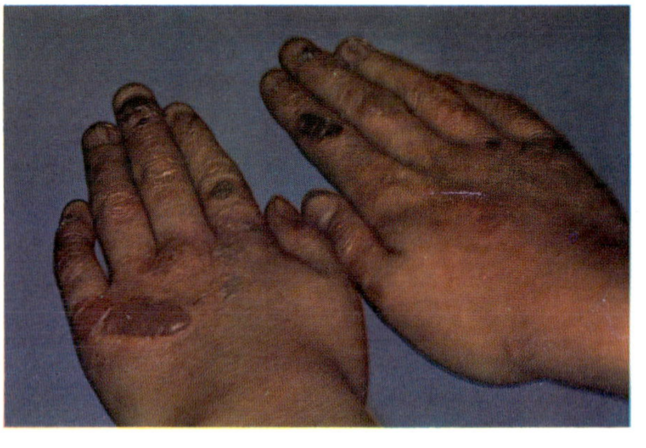

464 Epidermolysis bullosa dystrophica The bullous lesion on the dorsum of the left hand of this 8 year old boy is typical of the autosomal recessive variety of epidermolysis bullosa dystrophica. (See **357** and **474**)

465

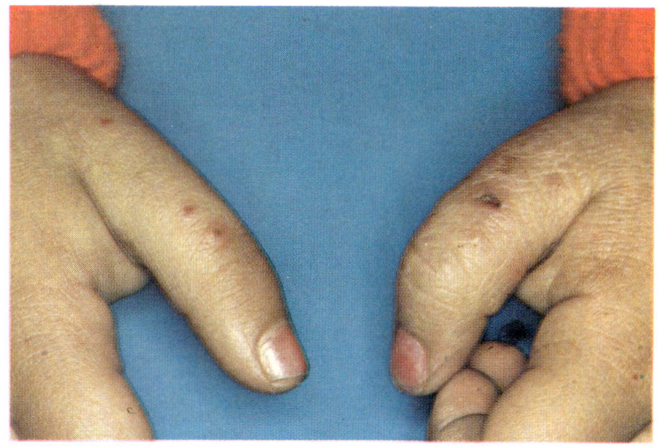

465 Acute herpetic infection The primary lesions of herpes simplex virus infection are seen on the dorsum of both thumbs in this young girl who was a bilateral digit sucker. The lesions were secondarily infected with coagulase positive Staphylococcus aureus. (See **328**)

466

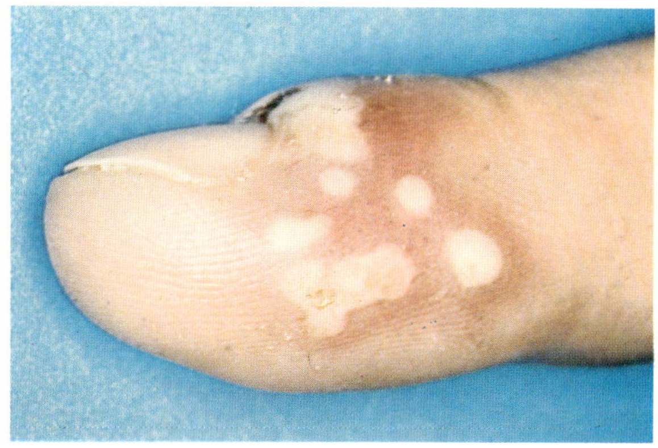

466 Acute herpetic infection (Herpetic whitlow) The vesicular lesions on the lateral aspect of the terminal phalanx of the index finger are evidence of a primary infection by the herpes simplex virus which is also involving the paronychial tissues of a paedodontist. Infections of this type can be transmitted from the oral cavity of an infected child patient.

467

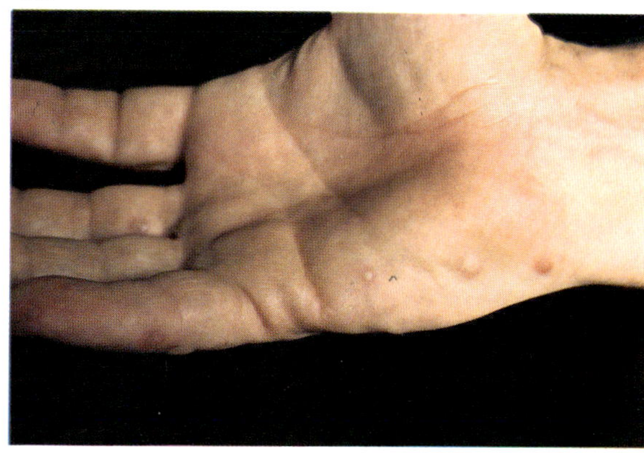

467 Hand, foot and mouth disease Papular, vesicular and ulcerative lesions affecting the skin of the left hand in an adult male whose five children were similarly affected by this Coxsackie virus infection. (See **346** and **475**)

468

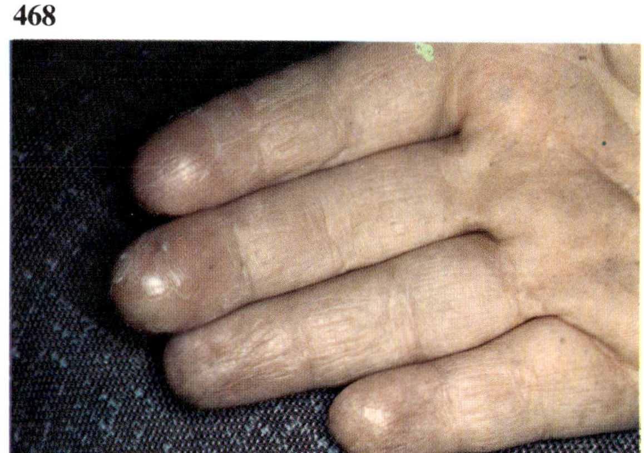

468 Exfoliative dermatitis Hypersensitivity to systemically administered penicillin caused the exfoliative dermatitis affecting the skin of the finger tips in this child.

469 Digit sucking This child has a curious persistent habit of sucking both the middle and index fingers of the left hand.

469

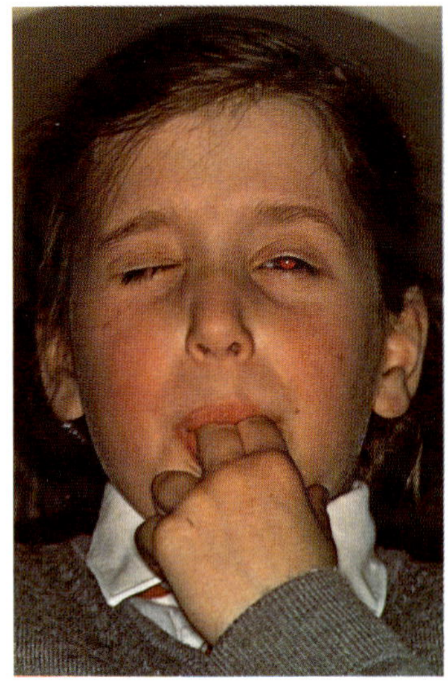

470 Hypertrichosis The dark brown hairs on the forearm of this 7 year old girl with hereditary gingival hyperplasia are up to 1cm in length. Similar hair is present on the lower limbs and down the middle of the back. (See **285** and **286**)

470

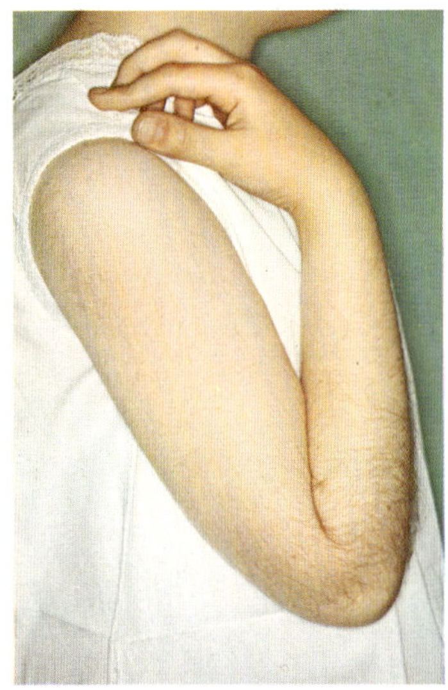

471 Thrombocytopenia Part of the generalised purpura in this adolescent is shown by the petechial haemorrhages into the skin of the upper arm. (See **298**)

471

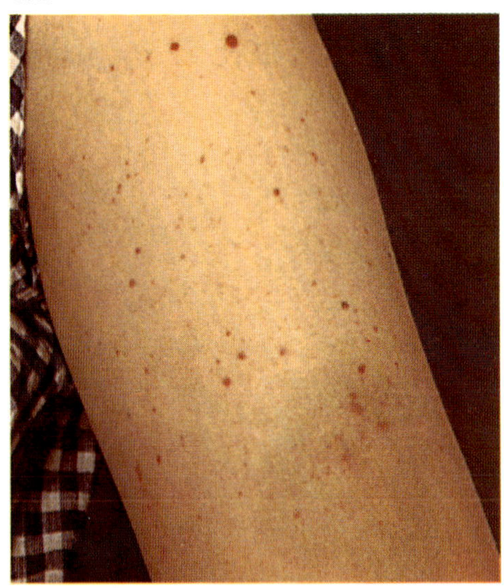

b. Lower limb

472

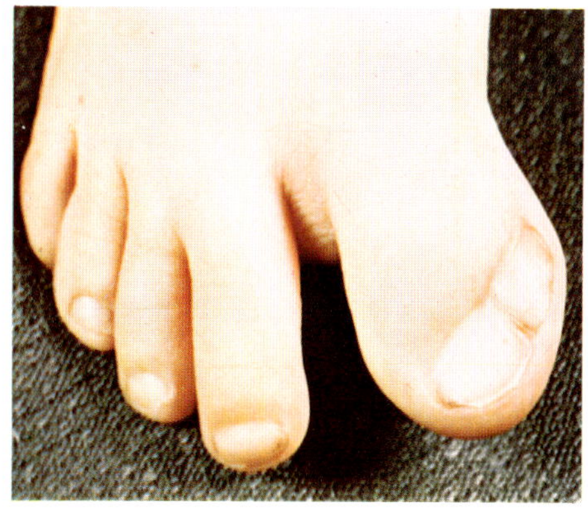

472 Orodigitofacial dysostosis (OFD syndrome) Curiously geminated hallux in child with the OFD syndrome. (See **366**, **410** and **411**)

473

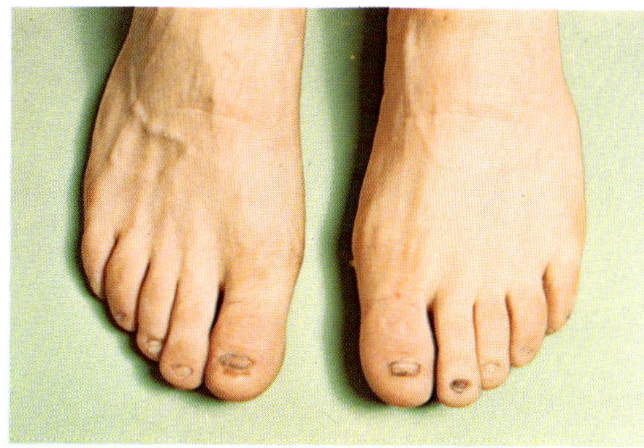

473 Tooth-nail dysplasia The dysplastic toe nails in this adolescent boy are associated with similar changes in the finger nails and a marked hypodontia in the permanent dentition. Conical deformity of incisor teeth is another feature. The anomaly is thought to be transmitted by an autosomal dominant gene and the affected tissues are limited to the nails and teeth.

474

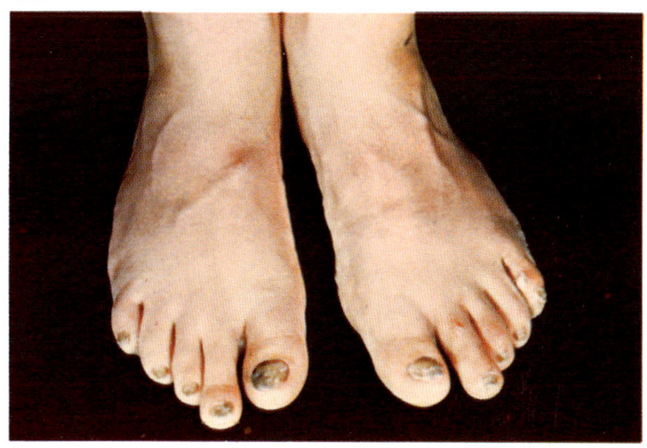

474 Epidermolysis bullosa dystrophica The dystrophic toe nails of a child with epidermolysis bullosa. The dark areas of staining are due to potassium permanganate treatment. (See **464**)

475

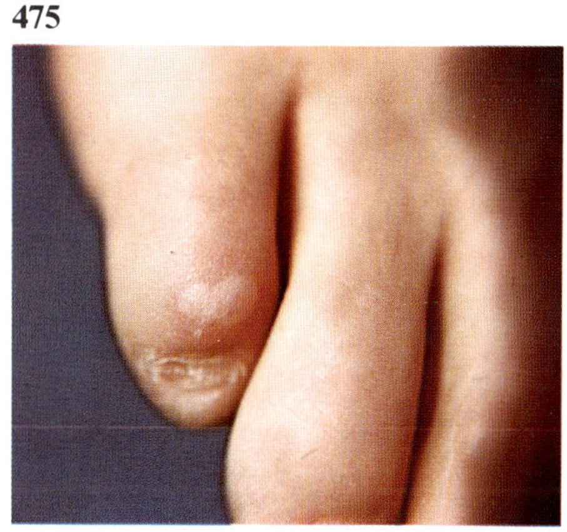

475 Hand, foot and mouth disease Large vesicular lesion on the dorsum of the fifth toe in the 5 year old daughter of an adult male with this acute virus infection. (See **346** and **467**)

476 Acrocephalosyndactyly (Apert's syndrome) The webbing of the toes in this child is a manifestation of Apert's syndrome in which craniostenosis is associated with syndactyly and other abnormalities. (See **7** and **378**)

476

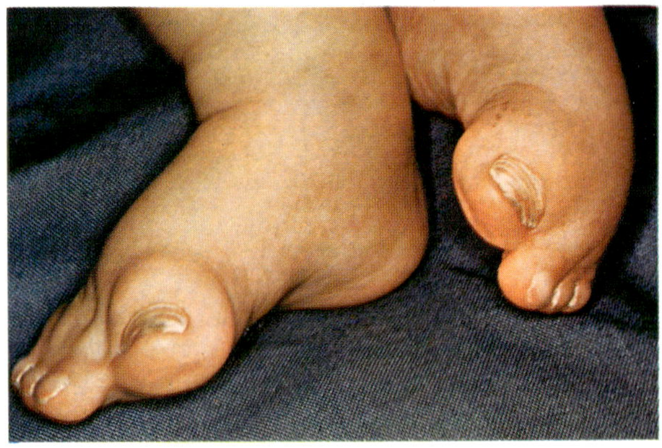

477 Osteogenesis imperfecta This radiograph shows the typical bony deformities seen in the pelvis and lower limbs of the severe infantile form of osteogenesis imperfecta. Note the characteristic bowing of the long bones and the healing fracture of the right femoral shaft. The defect is transmitted by an autosomal dominant gene (See **54** and **176**)

477

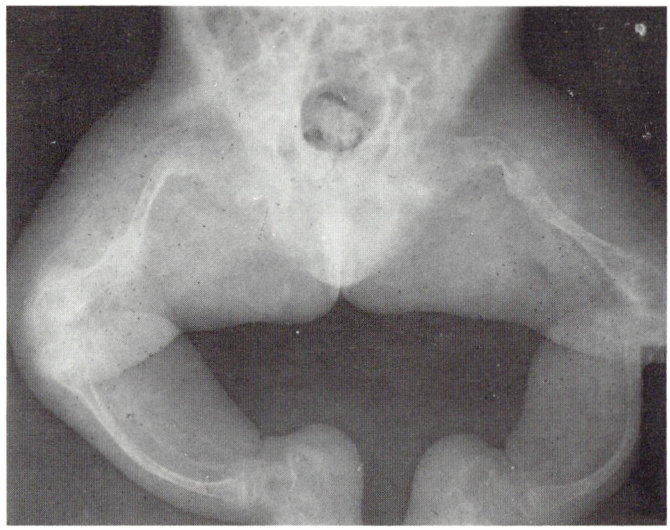

478 Vitamin D resistant rickets Deformity of the thighs and knees in a 4 year old boy with vitamin D resistant rickets. This defect of renal tubular phosphate retention is associated with hyperphosphaturia and hypophosphataemia. The abnormality is transmitted by an X-linked dominant gene. (See **141**, **142**, **177** and **178**)

478

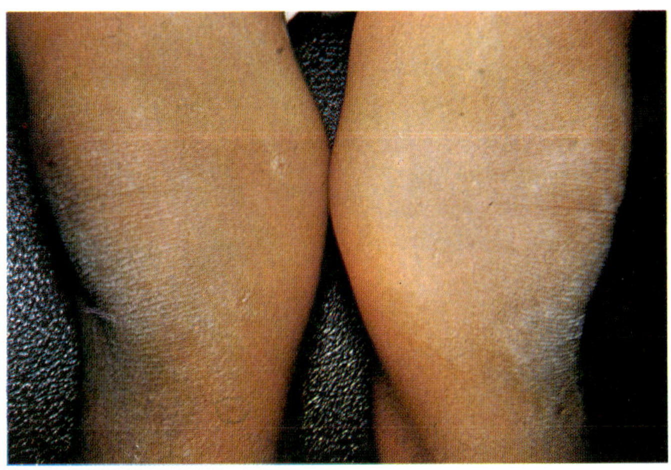

Index

Numbers refer to illustrations